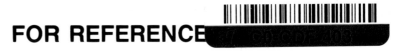

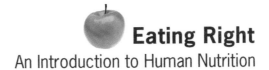

Eating Right
An Introduction to Human Nutrition

Basic Nutrition

Nutrition and Eating Disorders

Nutrition for Sports and Exercise

Nutrition and Weight Management

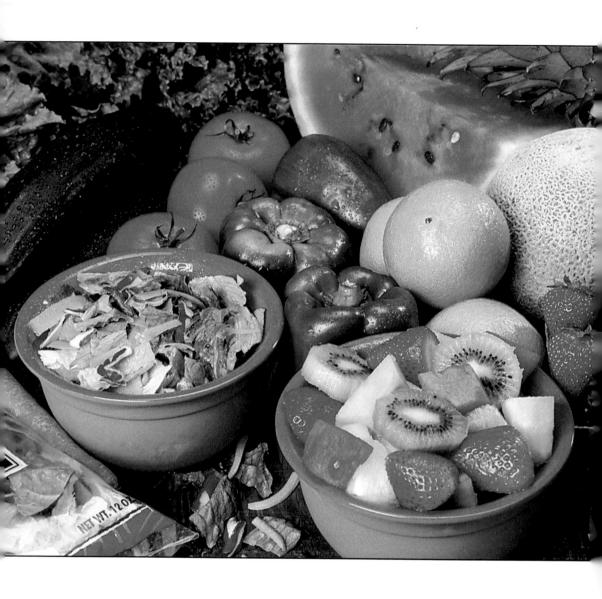

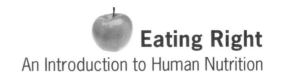

Eating Right

An Introduction to Human Nutrition

Nutrition for Sports and Exercise

Lori A. Smolin, Ph.D.
Mary B. Grosvenor, M.S., R.D.

Preface: Lori A. Smolin, Ph.D. and
Mary B. Grosvenor, M.S., R.D.

Introduction:
Richard J. Deckelbaum, MD, CM, FRCP(C)
Columbia University

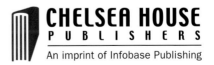

CHELSEA HOUSE
P U B L I S H E R S
An imprint of Infobase Publishing

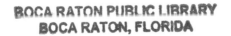

Frontispiece: Taking part in sports can be one of the most rewarding aspects of life. Proper nutrition, however, is vital to athletic performance. You should always include healthy foods like these in your diet.

Nutrition for Sports and Exercise

Copyright © 2005 by Infobase Publishing

Chelsea House
An imprint of Infobase Publishing
132 West 31st Street
New York NY 10001

ISBN-13: 978-0-7910-7853-2

Library of Congress Cataloging-in-Publication Data

Smolin, Lori A.
    Nutrition for sports and exercise / Lori A. Smolin and Mary B. Grosvenor.
        p. cm.—(Eating right)
    Includes bibliographical references and index.
    ISBN 0-7910-7853-1
    1. Nutrition—Popular works. 2. Athletes—Nutrition—Popular works. 3. Exercise—Physiological aspects—Popular works. I. Grosvenor, Mary B. II. Title. III. Series.
RA784.S598 2004
613.2'024796—dc22   2004009563

Text and cover design by Terry Mallon

Printed in the United States of America

Bang 21C 10 9 8 7 6 5 4

This book is printed on acid-free paper.

All links, web addresses, and Internet search terms were checked and verified to be correct at the time of publication. Because of the dynamic nature of the web, some addresses and links may have changed since publication and may no longer be valid.

About the Authors

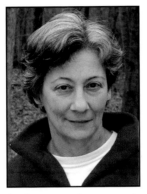

Lori A. Smolin, Ph.D. Lori Smolin received her B.S. degree from Cornell University, where she studied human nutrition and food science. She received her doctorate from the University of Wisconsin at Madison. Her doctoral research focused on B vitamins, homocysteine accumulation, and genetic defects in homocysteine metabolism. She completed postdoctoral training both at the Harbor–UCLA Medical Center, where she studied human obesity, and at the University of California at San Diego, where she studied genetic defects in amino acid metabolism. She has published in these areas in peer-reviewed journals. She and Mary Grosvenor are coauthors for two well-respected college-level nutrition textbooks and contributing authors for a middle school text. Dr. Smolin is currently at the University of Connecticut, where she teaches both in the Department of Nutritional Sciences and in the Department of Molecular and Cell Biology. Courses she has taught include introductory nutrition, lifecycle nutrition, food preparation, nutritional biochemistry, general biochemistry, and introductory biology.

Mary B. Grosvenor, M.S., R.D. Mary Grosvenor received her B.A. degree in English from Georgetown University and her M.S. in nutrition sciences from the University of California at Davis. She is a registered dietitian with experience in public health, clinical nutrition, and nutrition research. She has published in peer-reviewed journals in the areas of nutrition and cancer and methods of assessing dietary intake. She and Lori Smolin are the coauthors for two well-respected college-level nutrition textbooks and contributing authors for a middle school text. She has taught introductory nutrition at the community college level and currently lives with her family in a small town in Colorado. She is continuing her teaching and writing career and is still involved in nutrition research via the electronic superhighway.

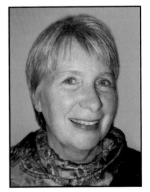

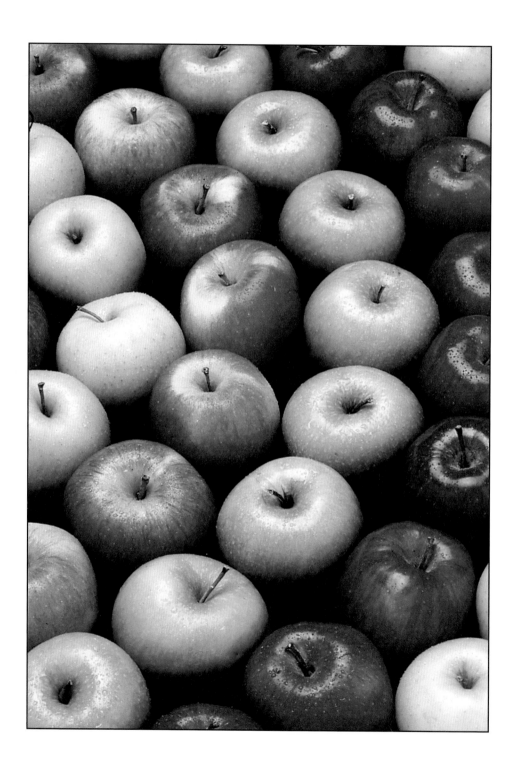

Contents Overview

Detailed Contents

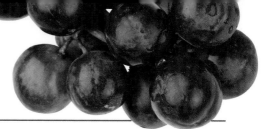

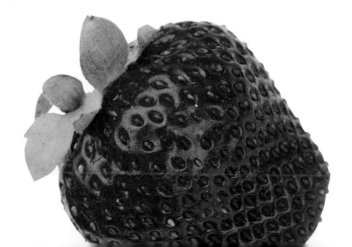

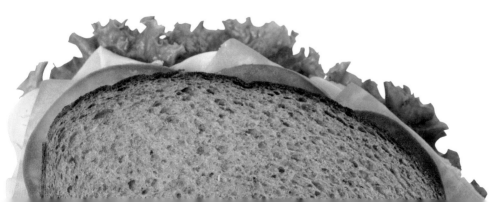

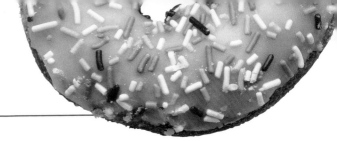

Preface

Lori A. Smolin, Ph.D.
Mary B. Grosvenor, M.S., R.D.

Fifty years ago we got our nutrition guidance from our mothers and grandmothers—eat your carrots, they are good for your eyes; don't eat too many potatoes, they'll make you fat; be sure to get plenty of roughage so your bowels move. Today, everyone has some advice—take a vitamin supplement to optimize your health; don't eat fish with cabbage because you won't be able to digest them together; you can't stay healthy on a vegetarian diet. Nutrition is one of those topics about which all people seem to think they know something or at least have an opinion. Whether it is the clerk in your local health food store recommending that you buy supplements or the woman behind you in line at the grocery store raving about the latest low-carbohydrate diet—everyone is ready to offer you nutritional advice. How do you know what to believe or, even more importantly, what to do?

Our purpose in writing these books is to help you answer these questions. As authors, we are students of nutrition. We enjoy studying and learning the hows and whys of each nutrient and other components of our diets. However, despite our enthusiasm about the science of nutrition, we recognize that not everyone loves science or shares this enthusiasm. On the other hand, everyone loves certain foods and wants to stay healthy. In response to this, we have written these books in a way that makes the science you need to understand as palatable as the foods you love. Once you understand the basics, you can apply them to your everyday choices regarding nutrition and health. We have developed one book that includes all the basic nutrition information you need to choose a healthy diet and three others that cover topics that are of special concern to many: weight management, exercise, and eating disorders.

Our goal is not to tell you to stop eating potato chips and candy bars, to give up fast food, or to always eat your vegetables. Instead, it is to provide you with the information you need to make informed choices about your diet. We hope you will recognize that potato chips and candy are not poison, but should only be eaten as occasional treats. We hope you will decide for yourself that fast food is something you can indulge in every now and then, but is not a good choice everyday. We hope you will recognize that although you should eat your vegetables, not everyone always does, so you should do your best to try new vegetables and fruits and eat them as often as possible. These books take the science of nutrition out of the classroom and allow you to apply this information to the choices you make about foods, exercise, dietary supplements, and other lifestyle choices that are important to your health. We hope the knowledge on these pages will help you choose a healthy diet while allowing you to enjoy the diversity of flavors, textures, and tastes that food provides and the meanings that food holds in our society. When you eat a healthy diet, you will feel good in the short term and enjoy health benefits in the long term. We can't personally evaluate your each and every meal, so we hope these books give you the tools to make your own nutritious choices.

Nutrition for Sports and Exercise is intended to give you an introduction to how the body uses food as fuel so that you can perform your best. It is important to provide your body with proper nutrition and remain hydrated for optimal performance, and those issues are discussed as well. We tackle some of the issues surrounding common nutritional problems that athletes may face at some point in their lives and dicuss dietary supplements commonly used by athletes to enhance performance. We also provide some guidance to choosing a healthy diet.

Lori A. Smolin, Ph.D.
Mary B. Grosvenor, M.S., R.D.

Introduction

Richard J. Deckelbaum, MD, CM, FRCP(C)
Robert R. Williams Professor of Nutrition
Director, Institute of Human Nutrition
College of Physicians and Surgeons of Columbia University

Nutrition is a major factor in optimizing health and performance at every age through the life cycle. While almost everyone recognizes the devastating effects of severe undernutrition, often captured on television during famines in underdeveloped parts of the world, far fewer people recognize the problem of overnutrition that leads to overweight and obesity. Even fewer are aware of the dangers of "hidden malnutrition" associated with inadequate intake of important vitamins and minerals. Unfortunately, there is also an overabundance of inaccurate and misleading nutrition advice being presented through media and books that makes it difficult for teenagers and young adults to decide for themselves what really is "optimal nutrition." This series, EATING RIGHT: AN INTRODUCTION TO HUMAN NUTRITION, provides accurate information to help people of all ages, and particularly young people, to acquire the needed tools and knowledge to integrate good nutrition as part of a healthy lifestyle. Each book in the series will be a comprehensive study in a different area of nutrition and its applications. The series will stress on many levels how healthy food choices affect the ability of people to develop, learn, and be more successful in sports, work, and in passing on good health to their families.

Beginning early in life, proper nutrition has major impacts. In childhood, good nutrition is important not only in allowing normal physical growth, but also in brain development and the ability to acquire new knowledge, both in and out of school. For example, proper dietary intake of iron is critical for preventing anemia, but just as important, it also ensures the ability to learn in the classroom and to be successful in sports or other spheres relating to physical activity. Given the major contribution of sports and exercise in improving health, it is easy to understand that nutrition truly is a partner with physical activity in promoting good health and better life outcomes.

Going into the adolescent years, many teenagers succumb to the dangers of fad diets—for example, undereating or alternatively overeating. Teens may not realize the impact of poor food choices upon their health, and, especially for girls, the risk that improper intake of vitamins and minerals will adversely impact their future families is very much underappreciated. As people mature into adults, nutritional practices have a major role in increasing or preventing the risk of major diseases such as stroke, heart attacks, and even a number of cancers. Thus, proper nutrition is an easy and cost-effective approach to achieving better growth and development, and later in markedly diminishing the chance of contracting many diseases.

Optimizing nutrition not only helps individuals but also has a major impact upon decreasing suffering and economic costs in families, communities, and nations. In the 21st century, individuals and populations will need to focus on at least three key areas. First, in promoting healthy lifestyles, nutrition needs to include a heavy concentration on diet and physical activity. Second, nutrition programs must focus on the realization that it is more important to work toward prevention rather than cure. Many of the early successes in nutrition focus on using nutrition as a treatment. We now know that improvement in nutritional status, which can easily be achieved, will have much more impact on preventing disease before it happens. Third, nutrition fits very well within the life cycle model. We know now that females who are healthy and fit *before* pregnancy are more likely to produce healthy babies and consequently healthy children. Conversely, women who have deficiencies of certain vitamins or unhealthy weights before pregnancy are more likely to have babies and children with significant health problems.

Developing countries now share the worldwide obesity epidemic. This series will help in the understanding that being overweight or obese not only changes physical appearance but also has a number of hidden dangers. For example, overweight and obesity are linked closely to rapid development of cardiovascular disease, type 2 diabetes, respiratory illnesses, and even liver disease and certain lung diseases. This "epidemic" must be fought by combined strategies using diet and physical activity. While many people today are striving to create more healthy lifestyles, they are unsure of how they should proceed. We feel that the books in this series will address these issues and provide the springboards for further thought and consideration about healthy eating.

This volume in the series EATING RIGHT: AN INTRODUCTION TO HUMAN NUTRITION presents the valuable information young people should know about nutrition and athletics. This book, together with the other editions in the series, will target specific areas to help readers achieve better outcomes for themselves and their families. With the knowledge to be gained through this series, we hope that each reader will be able to enhance his/her commitment to providing a better life for himself/herself and community.

Richard J. Deckelbaum, MD, CM, FRCP(C)
Robert R. Williams Professor of Nutrition
Director, Institute of Human Nutrition
College of Physicians and Surgeons
of Columbia University

1

What Is Nutrition?

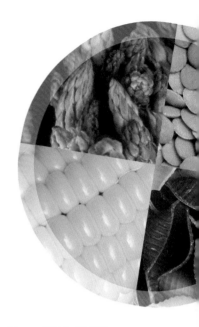

Nutrition is the study of all of the interactions that occur between people and food. It involves understanding which **nutrients** we need, where to find them in food, how our bodies use them, and the impact they have on our health. A study of nutrition also has to consider the social, cultural, economic, and technological factors that are involved in obtaining and choosing the foods we eat. Good nutrition is essential for health and athletic success. A diet that provides the right combination of energy and nutrients fuels exercise and allows for optimal performance. The effect of nutrition on exercise performance is greater for serious athletes, but even moderate exercise requires good nutrition. In turn, the amount and type of exercise an individual gets can influence his or her nutritional needs and overall health.

WE GET NUTRIENTS FROM FOOD

We don't eat individual nutrients, we eat foods. Food provides nutrients and also contains other substances, such as **phytochemicals**, that have not been defined as nutrients but have health-promoting properties. When we choose the right combination of foods, our diet provides all of the nutrients and other substances we need to stay healthy. If we choose a poor combination of foods, we may be missing out on some essential nutrients. Choosing a diet that provides all the essential nutrients can be challenging because we eat for many reasons other than to obtain nutrients. We may eat because we see or smell a tempting food; because it's lunchtime; because we're at a party; because we are sad or happy; because it's Thanksgiving, Christmas, or Passover; and for a multitude of other reasons. In order to meet nutrient requirements, we must understand what these needs are and how to choose a diet that provides them.

The Nutrients in Food

There are more than 40 nutrients that are essential to human life. We need to consume these nutrients in our diets because they either cannot be made in our bodies or they cannot be made in large enough amounts to optimize health. Different foods contain different nutrients in varying amounts and combinations. For example, beef, chicken, and fish provide protein, vitamin B_6, and iron; bread, rice, and pasta provide carbohydrates, folic acid, and niacin; fruits and vegetables provide carbohydrates, fiber, vitamin A, and vitamin C; and vegetable oils provide fat and vitamin E. In addition to the nutrients found naturally in foods, many foods have nutrients added to them to replace losses that occur during cooking and processing or to supplement the diet. Dietary supplements are also a source of nutrients. Although most people can meet their nutrient needs without them, supplements can be useful for maintaining health and preventing deficiencies.

What Do Nutrients Do?

Nutrients provide three basic functions in the body. Some nutrients provide energy. Others provide structure, and some help to regulate the processes that keep us alive. Each nutrient handles one or more of these functions, and all nutrients together are needed for growth, to maintain and repair the body, and to allow us to reproduce.

Energy

Food provides the body with the energy or fuel it needs to stay alive, to move, and to grow. This energy keeps your heart pumping, your lungs inhaling, and your body warm. It is also used to keep your stomach churning and your muscles working. Carbohydrates, lipids, and proteins are the only nutrients that provide energy to the body; they are referred to as the energy-yielding nutrients. The energy used by the body is measured in **Calories** or **kilocalories** (abbreviated as kcalories or kcals) or in **kilojoules** (abbreviated as kjoules or kJs). When spelled with a lowercase "c," the term *calorie* is technically 1/1,000 of a kilocalorie. Each gram of carbohydrate we eat provides the body with 4 kilocalories. A gram of protein also provides 4 kilocalories; a gram of fat provides 9 kilocalories, more than twice the kilocalories of carbohydrate or protein. For this reason, foods that are high in fat are high in calories. Alcohol can also provide energy in the diet—7 kilocalories per gram, but it is not considered a nutrient because it is not needed by the body.

The more calories you use, the more calories you need to eat in order to maintain your weight. If you increase the amount of exercise you get without increasing the amount you eat, you will lose weight. On the other hand, if you increase the amount you eat without increasing your exercise, your body will store the extra energy, mostly as body fat. When you consume the same number of calories as you use, your body weight remains the same—this is called energy balance.

Structure

Nutrients help form body structures. For example, the minerals calcium and phosphorus make our bones and teeth hard. Protein forms the structure of our muscles, and lipids are the major component of our body fat. Water is a structural nutrient because it plumps up our cells, giving them shape.

Regulation

Nutrients are also important regulators of body functions. All the processes that occur in our bodies, from the breakdown of carbohydrates and fat to provide energy, to the building of bone and muscle to form body structures, must be regulated in order to allow the body to function normally. For instance, the chemical reactions that maintain body temperature at 98.6°F (37°C) must be regulated or body temperature will rise above or fall below the healthy range. Many different nutrients are important in regulating **homeostasis** in the body. Carbohydrates help label proteins that must be removed from the blood. Water helps regulate body temperature. Lipids are needed to make regulatory molecules called **hormones**, and certain protein molecules, vitamins, and minerals help regulate the rate of chemical reactions within the body.

Getting Nutrients to Your Cells

The food we eat must be digested and the nutrients must be absorbed in order for them to function in the body. Digestion breaks food into small molecules and absorption brings these substances into the body where they are transported to the cells that need them.

The digestive system is responsible for the digestion and absorption of food (Figure 1.1). The main part of this system is the gastrointestinal tract, also called the GI tract. This hollow tube starts at the mouth. From there, food passes down the esophagus into the stomach and then on to the small intestine. Rhythmic contractions of the smooth muscles lining the GI tract help mix food and propel it along. Substances such as mucus and **enzymes** are secreted into the gastrointestinal tract to help with the movement and digestion of food. The digestive system also secretes hormones into the blood that help regulate GI activity. Most of the digestion and absorption of nutrients occurs in the small intestine. Absorbed nutrients are transported in the blood to the cells where they are needed. Anything that is not absorbed passes into the large intestine. Here, some nutrients can be absorbed and wastes are prepared for elimination.

How Your Body Uses Nutrients

Once inside body cells, carbohydrates, lipids, and proteins are involved in chemical reactions that allow them to be used for energy

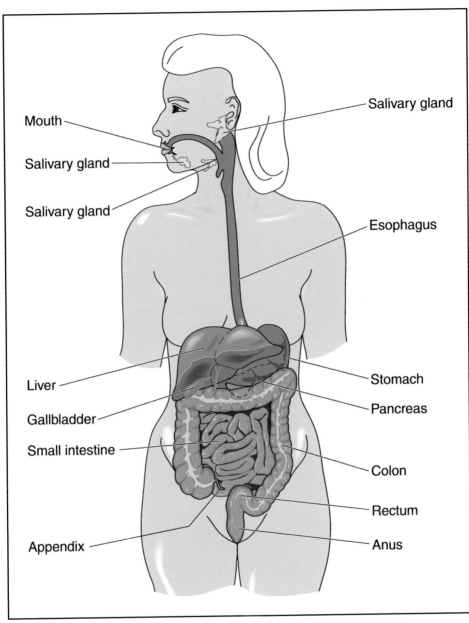

Figure 1.1 The digestive system consists of the gastrointestinal (GI) tract and accessory organs that aid digestion. Beginning when the person takes a first bite of food, the body starts the process of breaking down foods to put nutrients to work and preparing unneeded substances for elimination as waste.

or to build other substances that are needed by the human body. The sum of these chemical reactions, which occur inside body cells, is called **metabolism**. The chemical reactions of metabolism can synthesize the molecules needed to form body structures such as muscles, nerves, and bones. The reactions of metabolism also break down carbohydrates, lipids, and proteins to yield energy in the form of **ATP** (**adenosine triphosphate**). ATP is a molecule that is used by

---

FACT BOX 1.1

Bacteria In Your Intestine

Did you know that your large intestine is home to several hundred species of bacteria? You provide them with a nice warm home with lots of food and they do you some favors in return—if they are the right kind. These bacteria improve the digestion and absorption of essential nutrients; synthesize some vitamins; and metabolize harmful substances, such as ammonia, thus reducing levels in the blood. They are important for intestinal immune function, proper growth of cells in the large intestine, and optimal intestinal motility and transit time. A healthy population of intestinal bacteria may also help prevent constipation, flatulence, and gastric acidity. However, if the wrong bacteria take over, the result could be diarrhea, infections, and perhaps an increased risk of cancer.

How can you make sure that the right bacteria are growing in your gut? One way is to eat the bacteria. This is referred to as probiotic therapy. Live bacteria are found in foods such as yogurt and acidophilus milk and can be purchased as bottled suspensions or tablets. One problem with probiotic therapy is that the bacteria are washed out of the colon if you stop eating them. A second approach that can modify the bacteria in your gut is to consume foods or other substances that encourage the growth of particular types of bacteria. Substances that pass undigested into the large intestine and serve as food for these bacteria are called prebiotics. Prebiotics are sold as dietary supplements—but don't run to the store just yet. For most of us, eating a proper diet supports a healthy population of intestinal bacteria. Our understanding of how probiotics and prebiotics can be used to treat disease and promote health is still in its early stages.

cells as an energy source to do work, such as pumping blood, contracting muscles, or synthesizing new body tissue. The production and use of ATP will be discussed further in Chapter 2.

THE SIX CLASSES OF NUTRIENTS
The nutrients we need come from six different classes: carbohydrates, lipids, protein, water, vitamins, and minerals. Each class, with the exception of water, contains a variety of different molecules that are used by the body in different ways. Some classes of nutrients are needed in relatively large amounts, whereas others meet needs even when only tiny amounts are consumed. Carbohydrates, lipids, protein, and water are often referred to as macronutrients because they are required in the diet in relatively large amounts. Vitamins and minerals are referred to as micronutrients because they are needed only in small amounts.

Carbohydrates
Carbohydrates include **sugars, starches**, and **fibers**. Sugars are the simplest form of carbohydrate. They taste sweet and are found in fruit, milk, and added sugars like honey and table sugar. Starches are made of multiple sugar units linked together. They do not taste sweet and are found in cereals, grains, and starchy vegetables like potatoes. Starches and sugars are good sources of energy in the diet. Most fibers are also carbohydrates. Good sources of fiber include whole grains, legumes, fruits, and vegetables. Fiber provides little energy to the body because it cannot be digested or absorbed. It is, however, important for the health of the digestive tract.

Lipids
Lipids are commonly called fats. Fat is a concentrated source of energy. Most of the fat in our diet and in our bodies is in the form of **triglycerides**. Each triglyceride contains three **fatty acids**. Fatty acids are basically chains of carbon atoms. Depending on how these carbons are linked together, fats are classified as either **saturated** or **unsaturated**. Saturated fats are found mostly in animal products such as meat, milk, and butter. Unsaturated fats come from vegetable

oils. Small amounts of certain unsaturated fatty acids are essential in the diet. **Cholesterol** is another type of fat found in animal foods. Diets high in saturated fat and cholesterol may increase the risk of heart disease.

Protein

Protein is needed for growth, maintenance, and repair of body structures and for the synthesis of regulatory molecules. It can also be broken down to produce energy. Protein is made of folded chains of **amino acids**. The right amounts and types of amino acids must be consumed in the diet in order to meet the body's protein needs. Animal foods such as meat, poultry, fish, eggs, and dairy products generally supply a combination of amino acids that meets human needs better than plant proteins do. However, a vegetarian diet containing only plant foods, such as grains, nuts, seeds, vegetables, and legumes, can also meet protein needs.

Water

Water is an essential nutrient that makes up about 60% of the adult human body. It provides no energy but is needed in the body to transport nutrients, oxygen, waste products, and other important substances. It also is needed for many chemical reactions, for body structure and protection, and to regulate body temperature. Water is found both in beverages and in solid foods.

Vitamins

Vitamins are small organic molecules needed to regulate metabolic processes. They are found in almost all the foods we eat, but no one food is a good source of all of them. Some vitamins are soluble in water and others in fat, a property that affects how they are absorbed into and transported throughout the body. Vitamins do not provide energy but many are needed to regulate the chemical reactions that produce usable energy in the body. Some vitamins are **antioxidants,** which protect the body from reactive oxygen compounds like **free radicals.** Others have roles in tissue growth and development, bone health, and blood clot formation.

Minerals

Minerals are single elements. Some are needed in the diet in significant amounts, whereas the requirements for others are extremely small. Like vitamins, minerals provide no energy but perform a number of very diverse functions. Some are needed to regulate chemical reactions, some participate in reactions that protect cells from oxidative reactions, and others have roles in bone formation and maintenance, oxygen transport, or immune function.

HOW MUCH OF EACH NUTRIENT DO YOU NEED?

To stay healthy, adequate amounts of energy and of each of the essential nutrients must be consumed in the diet. The amount of each that you need depends on your age, size, sex, genetic makeup, lifestyle, and health status. General guidelines for the amounts of nutrients needed are made by the **Dietary Reference Intakes (DRIs)**. The DRIs were developed by teams of American and Canadian scientists who reviewed the current research and developed recommendations for the amounts of energy, nutrients, and other substances that would best meet needs and maintain health.[1] These recommendations are general guidelines for the amounts of nutrients that should be consumed on an average daily basis in order to promote health, prevent deficiencies, and reduce the incidence of chronic disease. The exact amount of any nutrient that an individual needs depends on his or her specific circumstances.

The DRIs

The DRIs include recommendations for amounts of energy, nutrients, and other food components for different groups of people based on age, gender, and, when appropriate, pregnancy and lactation.

The recommendations for energy intakes are expressed as **Estimated Energy Requirements (EERs)**. These can be used to estimate an individual's energy needs (see Appendix A). The recommendations for nutrient intakes include four different types of values. The **Estimated Average Requirement (EAR)** is the amount of a nutrient that is estimated to meet the average needs of the population. It is not used to assess individual intake but is designed instead for planning and evaluating the adequacy of the nutrient intake of population groups. The **Recommended Dietary Allowances (RDAs)** and **Adequate Intakes (AIs)** are values that are calculated to meet the needs of nearly all healthy people in each gender and life-stage group. These can be used to plan and assess individuals' diets. The fourth set of DRI values is the **Tolerable Upper Intake Levels (ULs)**. These are the maximum levels of intake that are unlikely to pose a risk of adverse health effects. ULs can be used as a guide to limit intake and evaluate the possibility of overconsumption. When your diet provides the RDA or AI for each nutrient and does not exceed the UL for any, your risk of a nutrient deficiency or toxicity is low.

What Happens If You Get Too Little or Too Much?

Consuming either too much or too little of one or more nutrients or of energy can cause **malnutrition**. Typically, we think of malnutrition

---

FACT BOX 1.2

How Much Does Activity Affect Energy Needs?

If you increase your overall level of physical activity, you need to eat more to maintain your weight. Using the EER equation shown below, you can calculate that a sedentary 16-year-old girl who is 5'4" tall and weighs 127 pounds needs to eat only 1,770 calories a day to maintain her weight. If she adds an hour of moderate activity to her day, she will be in the active physical activity (PA) category and will need to increase her food intake to 2,420 calories per day to maintain her weight. If she joins the soccer team and gets two hours of vigorous exercise at practice every day, she will be in the very active category and will need to increase her intake to 2,940 calories or more per day.

EER = 135.3 − (30.8 x Age in yrs) + PA [(10.0 x Weight in kg) + (934 x Height in m)] + 25

PA = sedentary 1.0, active 1.31, very active 1.56

as a deficiency of energy or nutrients. This may occur due to a deficient intake, increased requirements, or an inability to absorb or use nutrients. The effects of malnutrition reflect the function of the nutrient in the body and may appear rapidly or may take months or years to appear. For example, vitamin D is needed for strong bones. A deficiency of it causes the leg bones of children to bow outward because they are too weak to support their body weight. Vitamin A is needed for healthy eyes and a deficiency can result in blindness. For many nutrient deficiencies, supplying the nutrient that is lacking can quickly reverse the symptoms.

Overnutrition, an excess of energy or nutrients, is also a form of malnutrition. An excess of energy causes obesity. It increases the risk of developing diseases such as diabetes and heart disease. Excesses of vitamins and minerals rarely occur from eating food but are seen with the overuse of dietary supplements. For example, consuming too much vitamin B_6 can cause nerve damage, and excess iron intake can cause liver failure.

TOOLS FOR CHOOSING A HEALTHY DIET

Knowing what nutrients your body needs to stay healthy is the first step in choosing a healthy diet, but knowing how many milligrams of niacin, micrograms of vitamin B_{12}, grams of fiber, or what percent of calories should come from carbohydrates doesn't help you decide what to eat for breakfast or pack for lunch. A variety of tools has been developed to help you make these kinds of choices. Three of them—food labels, the Food Guide Pyramid, and the Dietary Guidelines for Americans—are discussed below.

Understanding Food Labels

Food labels are a tool designed to help consumers make healthy food choices. They provide readily available information about the nutrient composition of individual foods and how they fit into the recommendations for a healthy diet.

Almost all packaged foods must carry a standard nutrition label. Exceptions are raw fruits, vegetables, fish, meat, and poultry. For these foods, the nutrition information is often posted on placards in the grocery store or printed in brochures. Food labels must include both an ingredient list and a "Nutrition Facts" panel.

Ingredient List

The ingredient list indicates all of the ingredients used when preparing a food, including food additives, colors, and flavorings. The ingredients are listed in order of their prominence by weight. A label that lists water first indicates that most of the weight of that

---

FACT BOX 1.3

What Can You Believe?

Product labels and literature often make fabulous claims about the nutritional benefits of the products. Can you believe everything you read? How can you tell what is fact and what is fantasy?

Generally, the rule is, if it sounds too good to be true, it probably is. The following tips offer some suggestions for evaluating nutritional claims:

- Think about it. Does the information presented make sense? If not, disregard it.

- Consider the source. Where did the information come from? If it is based on personal opinions, be aware that one person's perception does not make something true.

- Ponder the purpose. Is the information helping to sell a product? Is it making a magazine cover or newspaper headline more appealing? If so, the claims may be exaggerated to help make a sale.

- View the claim skeptically. If a statement claims to be based on a scientific study, think about who did the study, what their credentials are, and what relationship they have to the product. Do they benefit in any way from the sale of the product?

- Evaluate the risks. Be sure the expected benefit of the product is worth any risks associated with using it.

food is water. You can look at the ingredient list if you are trying to avoid certain foods, such as animal products, or a food to which you have an allergy.

Nutrition Facts

The "Nutrition Facts" portion of a food label (Figure 1.2) lists the serving size of the food followed by the total calories, calories from fat, total fat, saturated fat, cholesterol, sodium, total carbohydrate, dietary fiber, sugars, and protein per serving of the food. The amounts of these nutrients are given by weight and as a percent of the Daily Value. Daily Values are standards developed for food labels. They help consumers see how a food fits into their overall diet. For example, if a food provides 10% of the Daily Value for fiber, then the food provides 10% of the daily recommendation for fiber intake in a 2,000-calorie diet. The amounts of vitamin A, vitamin C, iron, and calcium are also listed as a percent of the Daily Value.

In addition to the required nutrition information, food labels often highlight specific characteristics of a product that might be of interest to the consumer; for example, the label might advertise that a food is "low in calories" or "high in fiber." The Food and Drug Administration (FDA) has developed definitions for these nutrient content descriptors. Food labels are also permitted to include specific health claims if they are relevant. These are only permitted on labels if the scientific evidence for the claim is reviewed by the FDA and found to be factual.

The Food Guide Pyramid

The Food Guide Pyramid is a visual tool for planning your diet that divides foods into five groups based on their nutrient composition. Choosing the recommended number of servings from each group will provide a diet that meets the recommendations for an adequate diet that will help promote health and prevent disease. The shape of the Pyramid helps emphasize that the recommendations for the amounts of food from each of the five food groups (Figure 1.3). The wide base of the Pyramid is the Bread, Cereal, Rice, & Pasta

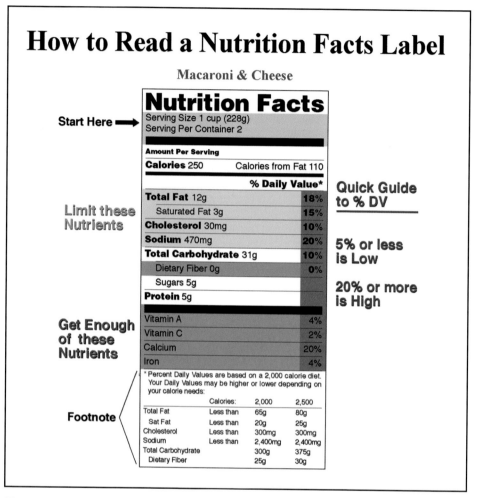

Figure 1.2 Standard nutrition labels like this one appear on all packaged foods. They provide information about the amount of calories, fat, sugar, and other nutrients that are in each serving of the packaged food. They can help you tell at a glance whether a particular food meets your nutritional needs.

Group; choosing between 6 and 11 servings of mostly whole grains forms the foundation of a healthy diet. The range of servings allows the Pyramid to be used by people with different calorie needs. For example, a 100-pound sedentary woman may need only 6 bread servings, whereas a 200-pound boxer may need 11 servings. The

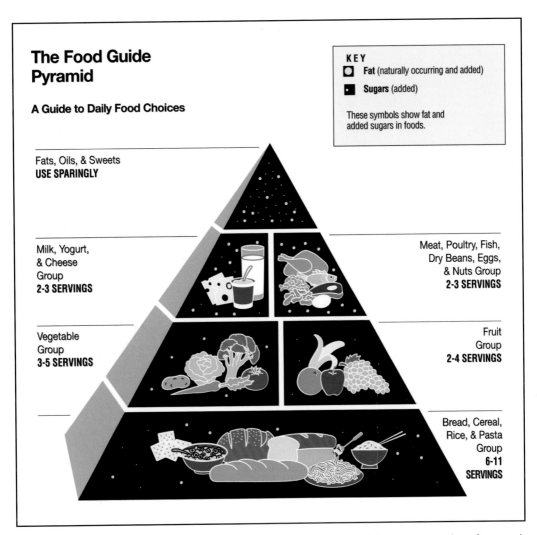

Figure 1.3 The Food Pyramid is designed to educate people about how many servings from each food group they should include in their diets. Although the recommended numbers of servings from each group are not rigid requirements, the Pyramid focuses on cutting fat out of our diets, since high-fat diets are a major problem in the United States.

next level of the Pyramid includes the Vegetable Group, of which 3 to 5 servings per day are recommended, and the Fruit Group, of which 2 to 4 servings per day are recommended. Health campaigns that promote "5-a-day" are encouraging people to meet the minimum daily Food Guide Pyramid serving recommendations of 3 vegetable and 2 fruit servings. The next level, where the decreasing size of the Pyramid boxes reflects the smaller number of recommended servings, comprises the Milk, Yogurt, & Cheese Group and the Meat, Poultry, Fish, Dry Beans, Eggs, & Nuts Group. Two to 3 servings a day are recommended from each of these groups. The narrow tip of the Pyramid includes a recommendation to use Fats, Oils, & Sweets sparingly in the diet.

The variety of foods in the Pyramid allows it to be useful as a guide for people from diverse cultures and lifestyles. For example, a Mexican American might choose tortillas as a grain, while a Japanese American might prefer rice; a vegetarian may choose beans from the Meat, Poultry, Fish, Dry Beans, Eggs, & Nuts Group, whereas someone else might prefer beef.

The Dietary Guidelines

The Dietary Guidelines for Americans is another useful tool that can help you choose a healthy diet. It is a set of recommendations on diet and lifestyle designed to promote health, support active lives, and reduce chronic disease risks. The guidelines are organized into 3 tiers: the ABCs for Good Health (Figure 1.4).

The first tier is called "Aim for Fitness." It includes two recommendations: "Aim for a healthy weight" and "Be physically active each day." These instructions are backed up by specific guidelines for body weight and activity levels.

The "Build a Healthy Base" tier offers four guidelines on choosing a variety of foods and handling these foods safely. It recommends that we let the Pyramid guide our food choices; eat a variety of grains, especially whole grains, daily; eat a variety of fruits and vegetables each day; and "Keep food safe to eat."

The last tier, "Choose Sensibly," recommends limiting intakes of certain dietary components. The first guideline, "Choose a diet that is low in saturated fat and cholesterol and moderate in total fat," reflects the understanding that diets low in saturated fat and cholesterol may reduce the risk of heart disease. The guideline to "Choose beverages and foods to moderate your intake of sugars" is based on

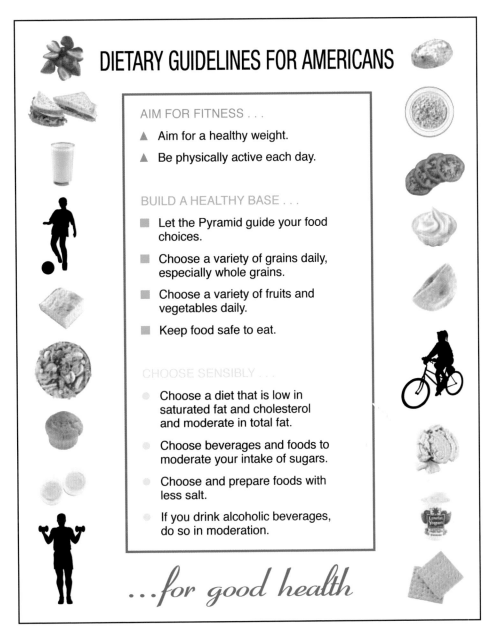

DIETARY GUIDELINES FOR AMERICANS

AIM FOR FITNESS . . .

▲ Aim for a healthy weight.

▲ Be physically active each day.

BUILD A HEALTHY BASE . . .

■ Let the Pyramid guide your food choices.

■ Choose a variety of grains daily, especially whole grains.

■ Choose a variety of fruits and vegetables daily.

■ Keep food safe to eat.

CHOOSE SENSIBLY . . .

● Choose a diet that is low in saturated fat and cholesterol and moderate in total fat.

● Choose beverages and foods to moderate your intake of sugars.

● Choose and prepare foods with less salt.

● If you drink alcoholic beverages, do so in moderation.

. . . for good health

Figure 1.4 The Dietary Guidelines for Americans can help a person choose a healthy and sensible diet. These guidelines suggest that people get enough exercise; choose a variety of different, nutritious foods; and limit their intake of certain food components, such as salt, sugar, and cholesterol.

the fact that the intake of sugar in the United States has been on the rise and may be increasing the incidence of chronic disease. "Choose and prepare foods with less salt" is based on research that indicates that a diet high in salt increases blood pressure in some

---

FACT BOX 1.4

How Healthy Is The American Diet?

A healthy diet should be based on whole grains, vegetables, and fruits, with smaller amounts of dairy products and high-protein foods and limited amounts of fats and sweets. As a population, Americans do not meet these recommendations. The Dietary Guidelines and the Food Guide Pyramid recommend that we choose whole grains rather than refined ones, but the average American consumes only one serving per day of whole grains. The Food Guide Pyramid recommends 2–4 servings of fruit but the average person eats only 1-2/3 servings each day and 48% of Americans don't consume even one piece of fruit daily. We also fall short of the 2–3 servings of dairy products recommended. Americans on average eat only 1-1/2 dairy servings daily and only 12% of teenage girls and 14% of women consume the recommended amounts.[a] In addition to the things we don't get enough of, we eat too much added sugar. The average American consumes about 64 pounds of sugar a year, or about 20 teaspoons a day, of added sugar. Much of this comes from soft drinks; Americans drink more than 13 billion gallons of carbonated drinks every year.[b] The typical American diet, along with a lack of physical activity, contributes to the development of chronic diseases, such as diabetes, obesity, heart disease, and cancer, which are the major causes of illness and death in the U.S. population. One estimate suggests that 14% of all premature deaths in the United States can be attributed to poor diet and a sedentary lifestyle. Recommendations for reducing disease risk focus on increasing activity patterns and choosing a diet that meets recommendations.

a. Cleveland, E., J.E. Cook, J.W. Wilson, et al. "Pyramid Servings Data from the 1994 CSFII data ARS Food Surveys Research." Available online at *http://www.barc.usda.gov/bhnrc/foodsurveys/home.html.*

b. "Pouring Rights: Marketing empty calories." *Public Health Reports 2000.* Vol. 115. New York: Oxford University Press, 2000, pp. 308–319.

individuals. The final guideline emphasizes the dangers of excess alcohol consumption.

CONNECTIONS

Human nutrition is the science that studies the interactions between people and food. Food provides nutrients, which are substances required in the diet for growth, reproduction, and maintenance of the body. There are six classes of nutrients. Carbohydrates include sugars, starches, and fibers. Sugars and starches provide energy, at 4 calories per gram. Fibers provide little energy because they cannot be digested by human enzymes and therefore cannot be absorbed into the body. Lipids are a concentrated source of calories in the diet and in the body, providing 9 calories per gram. They are also needed to synthesize structural and regulatory molecules. Proteins are made from amino acids. In the body, proteins can provide energy but are more important for their structural and regulatory roles. Water is the most abundant nutrient in the body. Water intake must equal output to maintain balance. Vitamins and minerals are needed in the diet in small amounts. They both have regulatory roles, and some minerals also provide structure. Consuming too much or too little energy or nutrients results in malnutrition. The Dietary Reference Intakes (DRIs) recommend amounts of energy and nutrients needed to promote health, prevent deficiencies, and reduce the incidence of chronic disease. The Daily Values on food labels, the Food Guide Pyramid, and the Dietary Guidelines for Americans present recommendations for choosing foods that will provide these nutrients.

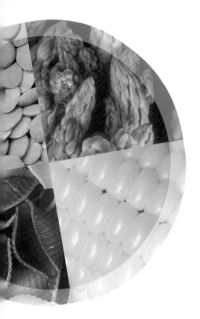

2

Energy for Exercise

Just as an automobile engine runs on energy from gasoline, the body runs on energy from food. Carbohydrates, fat, and protein in the foods you eat provide this energy, but before these nutrients can be used to power the body, they must first be converted to the high-energy molecule ATP (adenosine triphosphate). ATP is the immediate source of energy for all body functions. ATP supplies the energy needed to breathe, circulate blood, eliminate body wastes, and maintain body temperature. It also supplies the energy for muscle contraction, whether the muscles are needed to do your homework, walk to class, or compete in a track meet.

Small amounts of ATP and other high-energy molecules are stored in your muscles, but for muscle work to continue for more than a few minutes, additional ATP must be obtained from the metabolism of the energy-yielding nutrients. Which nutrients are metabolized and how much ATP they provide depends on whether oxygen is available in the muscle cells. The amount of oxygen available depends on the ability of the heart and lungs to deliver it to the cells.

ENERGY RIGHT NOW: ATP AND CREATINE PHOSPHATE

In order for your muscles to contract, ATP is needed immediately. In a resting muscle, there is enough stored ATP for you to use your muscles for about three seconds. As the ATP in muscle is used, enzymes break down another high-energy compound called **creatine phosphate** to replenish the ATP supply. The amount of creatine phosphate stored in the muscle at any time is also small. It will allow you to use your muscles for about an additional 8 to 10 seconds before it, too, is used up. So, during the first 10 to 15 seconds of exercise, the muscles use energy from the ATP and creatine phosphate that is stored there (Figure 2.1). At this early stage in exercise, your heart rate and breathing have not had time to increase, so the amount of oxygen at the muscle has not risen. Fortunately, no oxygen is needed to use the ATP or creatine phosphate stored in the muscle. High-intensity, short-duration exercise, such as a 100-meter dash, a 25-meter swim, or lifting a heavy weight, can be fueled almost exclusively by the energy from stored ATP and creatine phosphate. These sources are also important in any activity requiring brief bursts of maximal effort, such as driving for a layup in a basketball game, thrusting upward during a pole vault, or launching a shot put. However, sustaining exercise beyond an immediate burst and recovering from an all-out effort require additional ATP that is generated from the metabolism of carbohydrate, protein, and fat.

SHORT BURSTS OF ENERGY: ANAEROBIC METABOLISM

If you continue to exercise, the ATP and creatine phosphate in your muscles will be used up. Your muscles will then obtain ATP mainly from the metabolism of the sugar glucose. This can occur in the absence of oxygen through a process known as **anaerobic metabolism** or **anaerobic glycolysis**. Anaerobic metabolism predominates during the first few minutes of exercise, before your heart and lungs have been able to maximize oxygen delivery to the

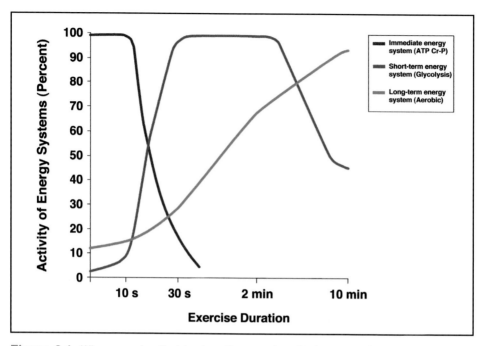

Figure 2.1 When exercise first begins, the muscles obtain energy from stored ATP and creatine phosphate. By 30 seconds into the activity, anaerobic pathways are operating at full capacity. Aerobic metabolism begins to make a significant energy contribution by about 2 minutes after the exercise has begun, and it is responsible for producing the energy needed for longer-term activity.

muscle. It is also important during periods of intense exercise, because oxygen cannot be delivered quickly enough to the cells to meet energy demands. Anaerobic metabolism can produce ATP very rapidly, but can only use glucose as a fuel and, therefore, cannot sustain exercise for very long.

Anaerobic metabolism takes place in the cytoplasm of the cell. The reactions break the 6-carbon sugar glucose into two 3-carbon molecules of **pyruvate** (Figure 2.2). By this process, each molecule of glucose generates two molecules of ATP, which are available to power muscle contraction.

The by-products of anaerobic ATP production—pyruvate and high-energy electrons—combine to form a molecule called **lactic**

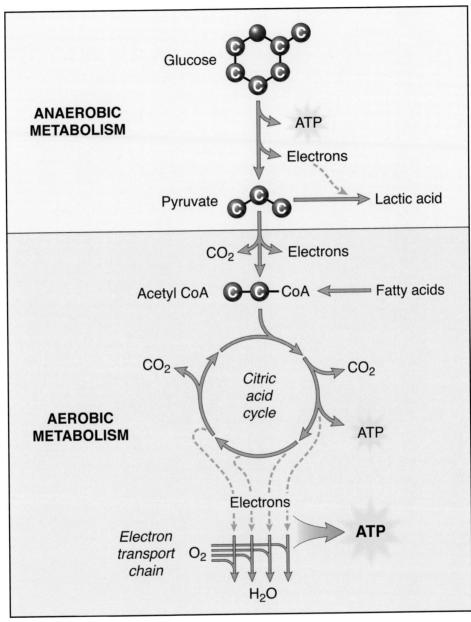

Figure 2.2 In the absence of oxygen, ATP is produced from glucose through anaerobic metabolism, which makes ATP quickly but inefficiently. When oxygen is available, aerobic metabolism can use both glucose and fatty acids to generate ATP. In this case, production is slower but more ATP is generated per glucose molecule.

acid. The lactic acid is transported out of the muscle for use in other tissues, such as less active muscles and the heart. However, if the amount of lactic acid produced exceeds the amount that can be used by other tissues, it begins to build up in the muscle and, subsequently, in the blood. This acid buildup causes an increase in the acidity of the muscle and contributes to fatigue and muscle pain.

ENERGY FOR THE LONG RUN: AEROBIC METABOLISM

If you are going to exercise for longer than a few minutes, the ATP used to fuel your muscle contractions will come primarily from the metabolism of carbohydrates and fat. How much of each source is used depends on the availability of oxygen at the muscles. When oxygen is available, ATP can be produced by **aerobic metabolism**. Aerobic metabolism can use glucose, fatty acids, and sometimes amino acids from protein for fuel. This process produces ATP at a slower rate than anaerobic metabolism but is much more efficient, producing about 18 times more ATP for each molecule of glucose. Once you have been

---

FACT BOX 2.1

Altitude Can Affect Athletic Success

When you go from sea level up into the mountains, you may feel lightheaded and short of breath. The is because the concentration of oxygen in the air is lower at higher altitudes. The reduction in oxygen can affect athletic performance. This fact was demonstrated at the 1968 Summer Olympic Games, which were held in Mexico City, located 7,349 feet (2,240 meters) above sea level. In short sprinting events, which rely mostly on anaerobic metabolism and therefore don't depend on the availability of oxygen, new records were set in almost every men's and women's race. But in distance events, the thinner air took its toll. Times were slower for running events over 800 meters (2,625 feet), where aerobic metabolism plays a more important role. The altitude also had greater effects on athletes who lived at sea level than those who were accustomed to higher altitudes.

exercising moderately for 2 to 3 minutes, aerobic metabolism takes over. By this time, your body has been able to increase the breathing and heart rate enough to supply the working muscles with more oxygen.

The reactions of aerobic metabolism take place in the mitochondria. When glucose is broken down by aerobic metabolism, the pyruvate produced by glycolysis is converted to a molecule called **acetyl CoA**. Acetyl CoA is generated by removing one carbon from pyruvate, leaving a 2-carbon molecule that combines with a molecule of CoA. When pyruvate is used to make acetyl CoA, lactic acid is not formed and the electrons released by glycolysis can be picked up by shuttling molecules and then used to generate ATP. When fatty acids are used as an energy source in aerobic metabolism, the fatty acid chain is first broken into 2-carbon units that form acetyl CoA. This process is called **beta-oxidation** and generates electrons that can be used to form ATP.

Acetyl CoA, whether from beta-oxidation or glucose break-down, enters the next stage of aerobic metabolism, the **citric acid cycle**. To begin the cycle, acetyl CoA combines with a 4-carbon molecule, oxaloacetate, which is derived from carbohydrate. The result is a 6-carbon molecule called citric acid. The citric acid cycle then removes 1 carbon at a time from citric acid until the 4-carbon oxaloacetate is re-formed. These chemical reactions produce 2 ATP molecules per glucose molecule and also remove electrons. The electrons are passed to shuttling molecules for transport to the last stage of aerobic metabolism, the **electron transport chain**. The electron transport chain involves a series of molecules associated with the inner membrane of the mitochondria. These molecules accept the electrons from the shuttling molecules and pass them from one to another down the chain until they are finally combined with oxygen to form water. As the electrons are passed along, their energy is trapped and used to make ATP (Figure 2.2).

Your body's maximum capacity to generate ATP by aerobic metabolism is called your **aerobic capacity** or **maximal oxygen**

consumption, also referred to as **VO_2max**. VO_2max is dependent on the amount of oxygen that can be delivered to and used by your muscles. A greater VO_2max allows you to perform more intense exercise without relying on anaerobic metabolism.

HOW MUCH STORED ENERGY IS AVAILABLE FOR EXERCISE?

Your body stores energy in a number of forms. As discussed above, there are small amounts of ATP and creatine phosphate available for immediate use in muscle. Once these are used up, stored carbohydrate and fat are used to regenerate ATP. In some instances, body proteins are also broken down to produce ATP.

Carbohydrate is stored as **glycogen** in both the muscles and liver. The amount of energy stored as glycogen is small compared to the amount stored as fat and the amount of protein available. There are between 60 and 120 grams of glycogen stored in the

---

FACT BOX 2.2

Who Has the Highest Aerobic Capacity?

Who has a greater ability to generate ATP by aerobic metabolism— a marathon runner or a cross-country skier? The answer is the cross-country skier. Elite cross-country skiers are the most powerful athletes in terms of aerobic capacity. Because the arms are used to pull and push on the ski poles, more muscle groups are engaged in skiing than in running. Therefore, the overall energy expended in skiing is as high as, or higher than, the energy expended to move the body the same distance on foot. Elite cross-country skiers have very high maximal oxygen uptakes; a VO_2max of 94 ml/kg/min was recorded for a male Norwegian Olympic champion cross-country skier. In contrast, competitive basketball and football players typically have VO_2max values that are about 60 ml/kg/min, healthy college-age men have VO_2max values of about 50 ml/kg/min, and poorly conditioned adults may have values below 20 ml/kg/min.

From: *Physiology and Psychology Performance Benchmarks.* Available online at
    http://btc.montana.edu/olympics/physiology/pb02.html.

Table 2.1   Available Energy in the Body

ENERGY SOURCE	PRIMARY LOCATION	ENERGY (CALORIES)*
Glycogen	Liver and muscle	1,400
Triglyceride	Adipose tissue	115,000
Protein	Muscle	25,000

*Values represent the approximate amounts in a 70-kg male.
Source: Cahill, G. F. "Starvation in man." *New England Journal of Medicine* 282 (1970): 668–675; Frayn, K. *Metabolic Regulation: A Human Perspective*. London: Portland Press, 1996, pp. 78–102.

liver. Stores are highest just after a meal. Liver glycogen is used to maintain blood glucose between meals and during the night. Eating a good breakfast will replenish the liver glycogen you used overnight. There are about 200 to 500 grams of glycogen in the muscles of a 70-kg (154-lb) person. Muscle glycogen is used to fuel muscle activity. Muscle glycogen levels can be increased by systematically consuming high-carbohydrate meals after depleting glycogen stores with exercise.

The body's fat reserves are almost unlimited. It is estimated that a 130-pound (59-kg) woman has enough energy stored as body fat to run 1,000 miles (1,609 km).[2] Most of this body fat is stored as triglycerides in **adipose tissue** located under the skin and around body organs, but small amounts are also located inside the muscle.

Protein that is used as fuel comes from the breakdown of muscle and other proteins in the body. Although protein is not stored specifically as an energy reserve, a considerable amount of protein can be broken down before body function is affected (Table 2.1).

Carbohydrate as a Fuel for Exercise

Glucose is the form of carbohydrate used by the muscles as a fuel source during exercise. The amount required depends on the frequency, intensity, and duration of the exercise, and the fitness level of the exerciser. The glucose may come from the breakdown of glycogen in the muscle or may be delivered by the blood.

How quickly muscle glycogen is used during exercise depends on the intensity of the exercise. High-intensity exercise relies on anaerobic metabolism, which uses glucose exclusively as a source of fuel. This glucose is derived mostly from muscle glycogen. Therefore, the more intense the exercise you perform, the more glycogen you use (Figure 2.3). Muscle glycogen depletion is one factor involved in the onset of fatigue during exercise. During lower-intensity exercise, the muscles can use fat for fuel, but some glucose is still needed. Some of this glucose comes from muscle glycogen and some is delivered in the blood. As exercise continues and glycogen stores decrease, glucose delivered in the blood becomes a more important source of carbohydrate.

The glucose delivered in the blood comes from liver glycogen stores, glucose synthesized by the liver, and carbohydrates consumed during exercise. Hormones released during exercise help ensure that blood glucose levels are maintained and can continue to supply glucose to body cells, including the muscle. For example, within seconds of the start of exercise, the hormones epinephrine and norepinephrine are released, and when blood glucose levels begin to drop, a third hormone, glucagon, is released by the pancreas. These hormones stimulate the breakdown of liver glycogen and the synthesis of new glucose by the liver.

When liver glycogen is broken down, glucose is released into the blood to help maintain blood glucose levels. As with muscle glycogen, liver glycogen can be depleted if exercise is intense or of long duration. When liver and muscle glycogen stores are depleted, the muscles must rely on glucose supplied in the diet and synthesized by the liver. The process of glucose synthesis is called **gluconeogenesis**. During exercise, gluconeogenesis occurs primarily in the liver. The amount of glucose that must be produced by gluconeogenesis during exercise depends on the extent of carbohydrate stores that are present before exercise

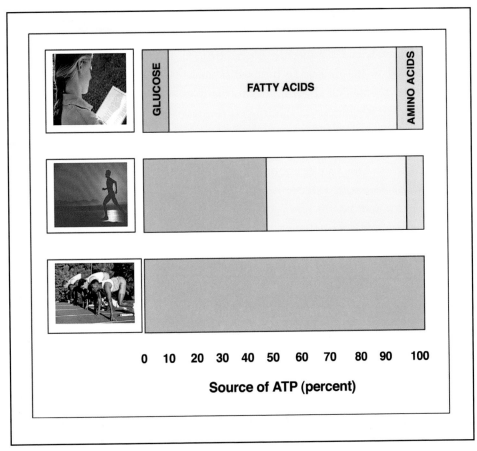

Figure 2.3 At rest, the muscles primarily use fatty acids as a fuel. Fatty acids are also an important fuel during moderate-intensity exercise. However, when exercise intensity is high, almost all of the energy for muscle contraction comes from glucose.

starts, the duration and intensity of the exercise, and how much carbohydrate is consumed during exercise.

Gluconeogenesis uses 3-carbon molecules, including lactic acid, alanine, and glycerol, to produce glucose during exercise. Lactic acid is generated by the anaerobic metabolism of glucose. Lactic acid produced in the muscle can travel to the liver and be converted back into glucose. Alanine is a 3-carbon amino acid generated from the release and breakdown of amino acids from the muscle. Glycerol is a product of triglyceride breakdown. When adipose tissue is broken down, the triglycerides yield three fatty acids and a molecule of glycerol. The fatty acids are transported to the muscle to be used to make ATP through aerobic metabolism. The glycerol goes to the liver, where it can be used for gluconeogenesis.

If you exercise for a prolonged period (3 hours or more), gluconeogenesis is a major source of glucose for your exercising muscles. Consuming carbohydrates in the form of beverages or snacks during exercise lasting 60 minutes or more can provide glucose and thereby spare glycogen, reduce the need for gluconeogenesis, and delay fatigue.

Fat as a Fuel for Exercise

Fat is a major energy source during exercise. It can only be used as an energy source when oxygen is available. In order to be used for energy, fatty acids inside the muscle cell must be transported into the mitochondria where aerobic metabolism occurs. The rate at which fatty acids can be used by the muscle depends on how quickly they can be delivered to mitochondria in the muscle cell. To enter the mitochondria, fatty acids must be activated and then transported across the mitochondrial membrane with the help of the amino acid **carnitine**. Once inside the mitochondria, beta-oxidation breaks fatty acids into 2-carbon units that form acetyl CoA. Beta-oxidation also releases electrons that are shuttled to the electron transport chain to generate ATP. The acetyl CoA can then combine with oxaloacetate to enter the citric acid cycle, where carbons are lost as carbon dioxide and electrons are shuttled to the electron transport chain to produce ATP and water.

Fatty acids used during exercise can come from adipose tissue, fat stored in muscle cells, fat consumed in the diet, or fat made by the liver. Most of the fat stored in the body consists of triglycerides found in adipose tissue. To be used by the muscle, the triglycerides must be broken down and the fatty acids transported in the bloodstream to the muscle. The breakdown of triglycerides in adipose tissue is stimulated by the rise in the hormone epinephrine that occurs as exercise begins.

Fat stored within the skeletal muscle, referred to as intramuscular fat, is also an important source of energy during exercise. This fat already exists in the muscle cells, so the fatty acids do not need to be transported in the blood. Higher-intensity **aerobic exercise** uses more intramuscular fat and individuals who are more physically fit may use more intramuscular fat because they can perform higher-intensity exercise without shifting to anaerobic metabolism.

Triglycerides consumed in the diet or made by the liver are a less important source of fatty acids for exercise. They are transported in the blood in particles called lipoproteins. At the muscle, an enzyme cleaves the triglycerides and allows the fatty acids to enter the muscle cell. Because people generally do not eat a large, fatty meal before exercising, the amount of energy obtained from blood lipoproteins is generally small.

When you perform moderate-intensity exercise (60 to 75% of VO_2max) for more than 90 minutes, carbohydrate stores will

---

FACT BOX 2.3

Which Bar Is Best?

Looking for a snack that will fit in your bike pack or pocket? A sports bar would be perfect, but deciding which one to choose may take longer than you think. There are many different types and they vary greatly in their nutrient composition and in the promises they make. If you're looking for an energy boost during your bike ride or day of skiing, you would probably do best with a high-carbohydrate bar, often called an energy or endurance bar. These have the sugar needed to prevent hunger and maintain blood glucose during a sporting event. Are they any better for you than a candy bar? Typically, they are lower in fat, higher in fiber, and contain more vitamins and minerals than a candy bar does. But are they as good as a meal? The answer is probably not, but if you can't fit a peanut butter sandwich and a banana in your pocket, they can be a good alternative.

be depleted and fat will become the primary energy source for muscle contraction. When fat is used as an energy source, glycogen stores are spared and exercise can continue for a longer period. A variety of dietary supplements, including carnitine and caffeine, have been suggested as **ergogenic aids** to increase the ability to use fatty acids as fuel. These will be discussed further in Chapter 6.

What Is the Role of Protein During Exercise?

Although protein is not considered a major energy source for the body, even at rest your body uses small amounts of amino acids for energy. The amount increases if your diet does not provide enough total energy to meet needs, if you consume more protein than you need, and if you are involved in certain types of exercise. The amino acids available to the body come from the digestion of dietary proteins and from the breakdown of body proteins. These amino acids can be used to synthesize new body proteins or other nitrogen-containing molecules. If the nitrogen-containing amino group is removed from an amino acid, the remaining carbon compound can be broken down to produce ATP or, in some cases, can be used to make glucose via gluconeogenesis.

Protein metabolism is affected by exercise intensity; high-intensity exercise increases the rate of protein utilization, whereas low-intensity exercise does not. Because amino acids from protein can be used to make glucose via gluconeogenesis, the availability of carbohydrate also affects the amount of protein used during exercise; protein becomes a more important energy source as carbohydrate stores are depleted. During exercise, amino acids can also be used directly by the muscles to generate ATP and to produce molecules needed for aerobic metabolism. When exercise is completed, amino acids are required to build and repair muscle.

The total amount of protein needed by the body is increased by strength training and endurance exercise. It is hypothesized that the additional protein used by strength athletes is needed to accelerate the rate of muscle protein synthesis and/or decrease the rate of muscle breakdown following strength exercise. Endurance exercise increases the use of amino acids both as an energy source and as a raw material for gluconeogenesis. The increased protein use in endurance athletes occurs because amino acids become an important source of energy when exercise continues for many hours. The glucose produced by gluconeogenesis helps maintain blood glucose levels during endurance activities. Additional protein may also be required to repair muscle damage caused by intense training.

Exercise Fatigue

When you exercise, ATP is produced by both anaerobic and aerobic metabolism. The contributions made by each of these systems overlap to ensure that adequate ATP is supplied to your muscles. The extent to which anaerobic metabolism is used affects how long you can continue exercising before experiencing **fatigue**.

Exercise fatigue occurs due to a combination of psychological, environmental, and physiological factors. Psychological factors such as mood can affect exercise performance; for instance, an athlete who is depressed may feel fatigued even before beginning an athletic event. Environmental factors such as temperature and humidity can also affect how quickly an athlete becomes fatigued. Physiological factors that affect fatigue include the depletion of liver and muscle glycogen and the accumulation of lactic acid. When athletes run out of glycogen, they experience a feeling of overwhelming fatigue that is referred to by runners as "hitting the wall" and by skiers and bicyclists as "bonking." Glycogen stores are depleted faster if anaerobic metabolism predominates. Anaerobic metabolism also results in the production of lactic acid. Lactic acid accumulation changes the acidity of the muscle, reducing its ability to contract. Lactic acid also inhibits the mobilization of fat from adipose tissue, forcing the muscle to rely more on glycogen, thus depleting it even faster. When exercise stops and oxygen is available again, lactic acid can either be metabolized aerobically in the muscle or carried away by the blood to other tissues to be broken down. After intense exercise, a mild cooldown, such as walking, may allow enough blood flow to the muscle to remove built-up lactic acid and prevent cramping.

If you exercise at high intensity, you rely heavily on the anaerobic metabolism of glucose. Your glycogen stores are used up rapidly and lactic acid accumulates, quickly causing you to fatigue. If you exercise at a lower intensity, you can continue exercising for longer periods before fatigue sets in because aerobic metabolism predominates. Aerobic metabolism is more efficient and uses mainly fatty acids for energy, sparing glycogen. However, even aerobic metabolism uses some glucose, so if you exercise long enough, your glycogen stores will eventually be depleted.

Your exercise conditioning also affects how long you can exercise before fatigue occurs. Exercise training causes physiological changes that increase VO_2max. A higher VO_2max allows you to perform more intense exercise without relying on anaerobic metabolism and, therefore, exercise can continue for longer periods without fatigue.

CONNECTIONS

The fuel needed to run the body machine is provided by the carbohydrates, fat, and protein in the diet. These nutrients are metabolized to produce ATP, the form of energy used to fuel body work. Small amounts of ATP and creatine phosphate, another high-energy compound, are stored in muscles. Once exercise begins, these fuels are used up quickly and additional ATP must be supplied by the breakdown of carbohydrates, fat, or protein. When oxygen is limited, as it is when exercise first begins and during intense exercise, ATP must be produced by anaerobic metabolism. Anaerobic metabolism can only use glucose as a fuel; it is a fast but inefficient way to produce ATP. It cannot sustain exercise for long periods because it quickly uses up glucose stored as glycogen and produces lactic acid that accumulates in muscles. Glycogen depletion and lactic acid accumulation both contribute to fatigue. When oxygen is available at the muscles, aerobic metabolism can proceed. Aerobic metabolism can use carbohydrates, fat, or protein to produce ATP. Aerobic metabolism does not produce lactic acid and, by using fatty acids as a fuel, it spares glycogen stores. Exercise that relies on aerobic metabolism can continue for longer before the athlete becomes fatigued. Exercise training allows athletes to perform at a higher intensity before anaerobic metabolism predominates.

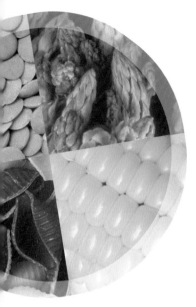

3

How Your Body Changes When You Exercise

Exercise changes the way the organ systems in your body function and interact. During exercise, some systems are stimulated to help the muscles do their work, while others are turned down to conserve energy. Your heart and lungs work harder to help supply oxygen to the muscles and eliminate waste products generated by body cells. At the same time, your digestive system slows down so that it does not burn energy that the muscles can use. These changes are all normal responses, whether you are a competitive athlete or just out for some weekend fun. The systems most affected are those involved in delivering oxygen to muscles and the muscles themselves.

GETTING OXYGEN TO MUSCLE CELLS

The respiratory system consists of the lungs and air passageways. The cardiovascular system includes the heart and blood vessels. Together, these two systems bring oxygen into the body and deliver it to tissues, including the exercising muscles.

They also help eliminate waste products from these same cells (Figure 3.1).

The Respiratory System: Take a Breath

When you inhale, the respiratory system brings oxygen into your body. Air enters by way of the nose or mouth and travels down the trachea to the branching air passageways in the lungs. In the lungs, oxygen from the air is transferred to the bloodstream and the waste product carbon dioxide is transferred from the blood to the air in the lungs for elimination. Most of the oxygen in the blood is bound to the protein hemoglobin found in red blood cells. Hemoglobin acts like a delivery truck that transports oxygen from the lungs to tissues throughout the body. Hemoglobin also transports carbon dioxide from the cells and delivers it to the lungs for elimination.

The Cardiovascular System: It Keeps on Pumping

The cardiovascular system includes your heart and blood vessels. It circulates blood, which transports oxygen and nutrients to all the body cells. The blood is pumped through the body by the heart. It is a muscular pump with two circulatory loops—one that delivers blood to the lungs and one that delivers blood to the rest of the body. The blood vessels that carry blood and dissolved substances toward the heart are called veins, and those that carry blood and dissolved substances away from the heart are called arteries. As arteries carry blood away from the heart, they branch out many times to form smaller and smaller blood vessels. The smallest arteries then branch to form capillaries, which are thin-walled vessels that are just large enough to allow one red blood cell to pass through at a time. The thin walls of the capillaries allow the exchange of nutrients and gases. In the capillaries of the lungs, blood brings carbon dioxide to be exhaled and picks up oxygen to be delivered to the cells. In the capillaries of the GI tract, blood delivers oxygen and picks up water-soluble nutrients absorbed from the diet. From the capillaries, blood flows into the smallest veins, which converge to form larger and larger veins for return to

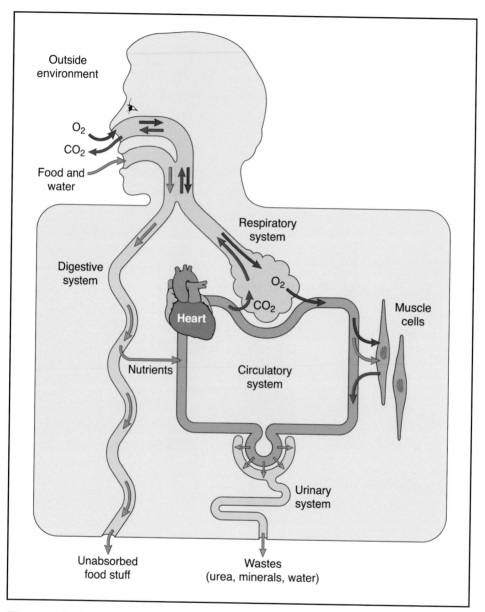

Figure 3.1 The organ systems of the body are closely interrelated. The digestive system takes in nutrients while the respiratory system takes in oxygen. Nutrients and oxygen are then distributed to the muscles and other body cells by the circulatory system. At the same time, the circulatory system also carries wastes from the cells to the lungs and urinary system to be eliminated from the body.

the heart. Therefore, blood that originates in your heart is pumped through your arteries to the capillaries of your lungs, where it picks up oxygen. It then returns to your heart via the veins and is pumped out again into the arteries that lead to the rest of your body. In the capillaries of your body, blood delivers oxygen and nutrients and removes wastes before returning to your heart via the veins.

HOW IS OXYGEN DELIVERY INCREASED?

When you exercise, your body uses more oxygen than it does when you are at rest. To make sure it gets enough oxygen, a number of adaptations occur during exercise to increase blood flow and the amount of oxygen delivered to the muscles.

Deeper, More Frequent Breaths

At the lungs, the increased need for oxygen causes a rise in the depth and rate of breathing. At rest, about 250 ml of oxygen is transferred from the lungs to the blood each minute, and about 200 ml of carbon dioxide moves in the opposite direction. During exercise, this exchange can increase 25-fold.[3] The increased rate of breathing ensures that the concentration of oxygen and carbon dioxide in the lungs remains within the normal range.

A Faster Heart

The total amount of blood pumped also increases with exercise. The amount of blood pumped by the heart during a one-minute period is called **cardiac output**. Cardiac output depends on heart rate, which is how fast the heart pumps, and **stroke volume**, which is how much blood it pumps with each beat. At rest, the heart rate of an average male college student is about 70 beats per minute and stroke volume is about 71 ml, resulting in a cardiac output of about 5,000 ml. During maximal exercise, the male student's heart rate would increase to about 195 beats per minute and stroke volume to 113 ml, resulting in a cardiac output of 22,000 ml!

Changing Blood Flow

Exercise also affects how the oxygen-rich blood is distributed. The volume of blood that flows to an organ or tissue, and, hence, the amounts of nutrients and oxygen that are delivered, depend on need. Blood vessels can either constrict or dilate to allow rapid redistribution of blood to meet an individual tissue's demand for oxygen, while maintaining blood pressure in the optimal range. As a person exercises, the blood vessels in active muscles dilate to increase the blood supply, while the blood vessels that supply the kidneys, liver, pancreas, and gastrointestinal tract constrict. When you are resting, about 24% of your blood goes to your digestive system, 21% to your skeletal muscles, and the rest to your heart, kidneys, brain, skin, and other organs.[4] When you engage in strenuous exercise, about 85% of blood flow will be directed to the skeletal muscles.

A Change at the Muscle Cell

During exercise, there is also a change at the muscle cells that increases the amount of oxygen picked up. This occurs because the metabolic reactions at the working muscle generate acids. The

---

FACT BOX 3.1

Training Boosts Cardiac Output

During maximum exercise, heart rate in both trained and untrained people is about the same—in young men, it is about 195 beats per minute. However, trained athletes are able to pump a great deal more blood with each beat of their heart because training has increased their stroke volume. During exercise, stroke volume is about 179 ml in trained men, compared to only 113 ml in untrained men. Therefore, a trained man's heart can pump 35,000 ml of blood per minute, compared to only 22,000 ml in an untrained man. This increased cardiac output raises the amount of oxygen that can be delivered to cells during exercise, allowing more efficient energy production via aerobic metabolism.

increase in acidity reduces the attraction between oxygen and hemoglobin, which results in an increase in the amount of oxygen released by hemoglobin and picked up by the muscle.

HOW DO MUSCLES WORK?

The human body has three types of muscles. The type used to propel you up a flight of stairs, around a track, or through the swimming pool is called **skeletal muscle**. Skeletal muscles are attached to the bones of the skeleton and are under voluntary control, meaning that they move when you want them to move. They are responsible for all voluntary movement. There are more than 600 skeletal muscles in the body. During exercise, the activity of the skeletal muscles increases greatly.

The heart is made up of **cardiac muscle**. Unlike skeletal muscle, cardiac muscle is not under voluntary control. Your heart continues to beat whether you are aware of it or not. Internal signals adjust your heart rate as needed to meet the oxygen demands of the body tissues and to maintain homeostasis. During exercise, your heart works harder to deliver more oxygen-rich blood to your muscles.

The third type of muscle is called **smooth muscle**. It lines the vessels that deliver blood to body cells, the air passageways through which air passes on its way in and out of the lungs, and the walls of glands and other organs. This type of muscle is also considered involuntary muscle because the contractions and relaxations of such muscles are not under conscious control. Smooth muscle plays an important role during exercise. For example, it is the smooth muscles in the blood vessels that constrict or relax to distribute blood to the tissues in need.

The mechanism that causes contraction is the same in skeletal, cardiac, and smooth muscle. Muscles are made up of bundles of muscle cells, referred to as muscle fibers. Inside each muscle fiber are hundreds to thousands of rod-like structures called **myofibrils**, which are responsible for muscle contraction. Each myofibril is made up of even smaller structures called filaments. There are two types of filaments—thick and thin. Thick filaments are made up of the protein **myosin** and thin filaments are made up of long chains of the protein **actin**. In order for a muscle to contract, myosin must attach to actin and rotate, causing the thin and thick filaments to slide past each other. This sliding increases the amount of overlap of the muscle filaments and shortens or contracts the muscle. This process requires ATP (Figure 3.2).

Muscles for Strength, Power, and Endurance

There are three major aspects of muscle performance: strength, power, and endurance.[5] Muscle strength is the maximum force that a muscle can develop. Strength is directly related to muscle size; increasing muscle size increases strength. Power refers to how fast the muscle can develop its maximum strength. It depends on both strength and speed. Muscle power gives you great acceleration, so it is important in short speed events like sprint running and sprint cycling and in sports like basketball where jumping is important. Increasing muscle power will increase the speed of the pitcher's fastball. Muscle endurance is the capacity to generate or sustain maximal force repeatedly. It is important for athletes involved in long events such as marathons, distance cycling, or triathlons.

The level of strength, power, and endurance that your muscles are able to achieve is due in part to the distribution of different types of fibers within your muscles. There are two primary types of muscle fibers: slow twitch and fast twitch. They differ in their speed of action—fast twitch fibers can contract as much as 10 times faster than slow twitch fibers can. Fast twitch fibers have a greater capacity for ATP production via anaerobic metabolism. Fast twitch fibers are important during activities that require changes of pace or stop-and-go movement, as in basketball, soccer, and hockey. These fibers are also needed during an all-out effort requiring rapid and powerful movements, such as running a 100-meter dash. Having a high proportion of fast twitch muscle fibers is an asset in time-limited activities such as sprinting, but fast twitch fibers tire quickly. In contrast,

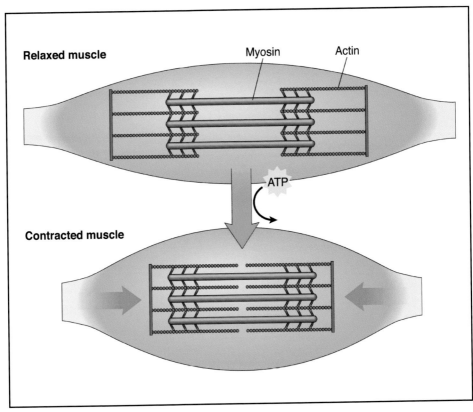

Relaxed muscle   Myosin   Actin

ATP

Contracted muscle

Figure 3.2 When muscles contract, actin and myosin filaments slide past one another to shorten the muscle. ATP provides the energy that allows a muscle contraction to take place.

slow twitch fibers develop force slowly, but can maintain contractions longer. They generate ATP primarily through aerobic metabolism. The slow twitch muscles contain more mitochondria, the cellular organelles in which aerobic metabolism occurs. They also contain more myoglobin, a protein that stores oxygen in the muscle. This makes them more efficient at using oxygen to generate ATP without lactic acid buildup. With sufficient oxygen, slow twitch muscles can maintain muscular activity for prolonged periods of time. The body relies on slow twitch fibers during low-intensity endurance events, such as long bike rides, and during everyday activities like walking. Most activities rely on a mixture of fast twitch and slow twitch fibers. For example, both would play a role in relatively short, higher-intensity endurance events such as a kilometer run or a 400-meter swim. During highly explosive events such as the 100-meter dash, the body relies mainly on fast twitch muscle fibers.

Genetics largely determines the types of muscle fibers you have. Most people tend to have an equal distribution of both fiber types. This is not true for certain elite athletes, though. Olympic sprinters have been shown to possess about 80% fast twitch fibers, whereas those who excel in long-distance runs like marathons may have 80% slow twitch fibers.[6] It is not clear whether training can change the distribution of fiber types within an individual.

THE EFFECTS OF EXERCISE TRAINING

The availability of oxygen in muscle cells is determined by how quickly the heart can pump blood from the lungs, where it picks

---

FACT BOX 3.2

What Is the Difference Between White and Dark Meat?

Ever wonder why a turkey leg has dark meat and a breast has white meat? The reason is that they are made up of different types of skeletal muscle fibers. The dark meat is found in the legs of chickens and turkeys. These birds are constantly walking but not very quickly. Therefore, their leg muscles need to be able to perform long, slow, continuous activity. These muscles are made up mostly of slow twitch fibers. The breast muscles of these birds, on the other hand, are needed for flight. The birds only fly in quick bursts to escape danger. The breast muscles, therefore, consist of fast twitch fibers that get them off the ground quickly. The dark meat is darker in color because the slow twitch muscle is richer in mitochondria, which contain red-pigmented compounds, and in red-colored myoglobin to support aerobic metabolism. The white meat muscles are used for quick bursts of anaerobic metabolism and have fewer blood vessels, fewer mitochondria, and less myoglobin.

up oxygen, to the muscle cells; by the amount of hemoglobin in the blood, which determines how much oxygen the blood can carry; and by how much oxygen can be used at the muscle cell. Training, by repeated bouts of exercise, causes physiological changes that increase the body's ability to deliver and use oxygen as well as the strength and endurance of muscles. Training also improves the ability to dissipate heat, allowing better performance in a hot environment.

What Does Aerobic Training Do?

Aerobic exercise is exercise performed at an intensity that increases the heart rate but still relies on aerobic metabolism. An activity is generally considered aerobic if it is low enough in intensity that you can carry on a conversation while exercising but high enough in intensity that you cannot sing. Aerobic training causes physiological changes in the cardiovascular system and the muscles that increase your aerobic capacity or VO_2max. This increases your overall endurance.

Regular aerobic exercise strengthens heart muscle and increases stroke volume. When the stroke volume is increased, the heart can deliver more blood with each beat. This increases oxygen delivery during exercise. At rest, the heart does not need to beat as many times to deliver the same amount of blood. Therefore, the more fit you are, the lower your resting heart rate and the more activity you can perform before reaching your maximum heart rate, which is the maximum number of beats per minute that the heart can attain.

Aerobic training also causes other changes that increase VO_2max. It raises the number of capillaries in the muscles so that blood is delivered to muscles more efficiently. It increases the total volume of blood and the number of red blood cells, making the total amount of hemoglobin greater, allowing more oxygen to be transported. Aerobic training also causes changes at the cellular level that improve the ability of the muscle cell to use aerobic metabolism. There is an increase in the number and size of mitochondria in the muscle cells as well as a boost in the activity of enzymes within the mitochondria needed for aerobic metabolism and fatty acid breakdown. There is a rise in the availability and transport of fatty acids to the mitochondria and an increase in triglyceride storage and oxidation in the muscle. These changes build up the cell's capacity to burn fatty acids to produce ATP. The use of fatty acids spares glycogen, which delays the onset of fatigue. Training also augments the ability to store glycogen. Because trained athletes store more glycogen and use it more slowly, they can sustain aerobic exercise for longer periods at higher intensities than untrained individuals can. A conditioned athlete can also exercise at a higher percentage of his or her VO_2max before lactic acid begins to accumulate.

FACT BOX 3.3

How Low Does Your Heart Go?

What is your resting heart rate? To find out, measure your pulse when you first wake up in the morning, before your feet even hit the floor. Have a watch handy, then find your pulse. You can find it either in your wrist or at the carotid artery in your neck. Use your index and middle fingers to count the beats. Don't use your thumb; it has a light pulse of its own that can cause confusion. If you are patient, count the number of beats in 60 seconds; if not, you can use a shortcut by counting the beats in 10 seconds and multiplying by 6. For example, if you count 11 beats in 10 seconds, your resting heart rate is 66.

The average resting heart rate is 66–72 beats per minute (bpm). A well-trained endurance athlete may have a resting heart rate of 40 bpm. Tennis great Bjorn Borg had a resting heart rate of 35 bpm. The lowest resting heart rate on record is 28 bpm, recorded for Spanish cyclist Miguel Indurain. But don't lose heart—ability and performance do not directly correlate with resting heart rate. Genetics accounts for much of your resting heart rate. For example, marathon superstar Frank Shorter had a resting heart rate of 75 beats per minute. Regardless of your genes and your current resting heart rate, getting in better shape reduces your resting heart rate, making your heart more efficient.

What Does Resistance Training Do?

Resistance training, often called strength training or weight training, involves using your muscles to push against a force. The most common type of resistance training is weight lifting. It can improve muscle strength, power, and overall endurance. Even elderly, sedentary individuals can increase muscle strength dramatically with weight training. The body adapts to perform the task demanded, whether that task is to lift a heavier weight, stretch a millimeter farther, or continue lifting for a few minutes longer. When a muscle is exercised, the stress or overload causes the muscle to adapt by increasing in size and strength—a process referred to as **hypertrophy**. By progressively increasing the amount or intensity of exercise at each exercise session, the muscle slowly hypertrophies. The greater the increase in exercise, the larger the effect of the training. By increasing the strength of muscles, resistance training can also improve the power of muscles. Gains in muscle endurance occur when muscle strength is increased, when cardiovascular performance is improved by aerobic training, and when diet is optimized.

When a muscle is not used due to a lapse in training, an injury, or illness, it becomes smaller and weaker. This process is called **atrophy**. For example, when an individual is bedridden and unable to move about, the muscles atrophy. Once the individual is up and active again, the muscles regain their strength and size.

CONNECTIONS

Exercise changes the way the organ systems in the body function and interact. During exercise, the respiratory and cardiovascular systems work harder to deliver additional fuel and oxygen to the muscles and to remove carbon dioxide and other wastes. Cardiac output increases and the blood vessels in the muscles dilate to improve blood delivery. Muscle performance depends on strength, power, and endurance. These parameters are due in part to the distribution of fast twitch and slow twitch muscle fibers. Fast twitch fibers have a greater capacity to use anaerobic metabolism, whereas slow twitch fibers generate ATP primarily through aerobic metabolism. Aerobic training causes changes that increase aerobic capacity (VO_2max), which is the maximum capacity to generate ATP by aerobic metabolism. Training boosts oxygen delivery by strengthening the heart muscle and raising stroke volume, the number of capillaries at the muscle, total blood volume, and the number of red blood cells. At the muscle, aerobic training increases the number and size of mitochondria. Resistance training, such as lifting weights, can improve muscle strength and power. When a muscle is stressed by a heavy weight, it adapts by increasing in size

---

FACT BOX 3.4

Use It or Lose It: Muscles in Space

You have probably heard the expression "Use it or lose it." Well, this motto is particularly important for astronauts. In orbit, where astronauts are free of the force of gravity, they do not need to use their muscles to stand and walk and support themselves. As a result, their muscles atrophy very quickly, getting smaller and weaker. The leg and back muscles, which are used to resist gravity on Earth, are particularly affected by a lack of gravity. When astronauts return to Earth, their decreased muscle mass and strength leads to difficulties in performing routine activities.

In order to prevent muscle loss while in space, astronauts must maintain a strict exercise program. They exercise on specially designed equipment that simulates the effect of working against the force of gravity. Sometimes they use stationary bikes, which provide good cardiovascular exercise. They also use treadmills; these are more cumbersome to use because the astronauts must be strapped down to add resistance and to keep them from floating away from the machine.

Despite rigid exercise routines, astronauts lose muscle mass during space travel. Fortunately, this is temporary, at least for short-duration flights. Whether or not muscle atrophy from long-duration space travel is reversible is currently under investigation. Understanding why muscle atrophy occurs could help us understand the muscle wasting that occurs in people who are bedridden and in all of us as we grow old.

and strength—a process referred to as hypertrophy. In contrast, muscles that are not used get smaller and weaker, which is referred to as atrophy. Improvements in overall endurance occur when muscle strength is increased and cardiovascular performance is improved by aerobic training.

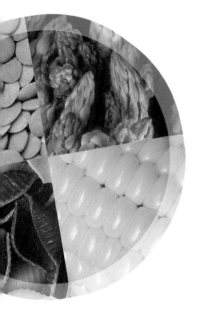

4

What Should Athletes Eat?

For most people who exercise, meals require no special planning beyond what is needed to consume a healthy diet. For competitive athletes, however, the right food choices may add or take away the extra seconds that can mean victory or defeat. An athlete's diet must provide enough calories from appropriate sources to fuel activity; adequate protein to build, maintain, and repair tissues; ample fluid to balance losses; and sufficient vitamins and minerals to allow for the utilization of the energy-yielding nutrients and optimization of other physiological processes. With all of these factors considered, the main differences between the diet of an athlete and that of a casual exerciser are the needs for additional energy to fuel physical activity and extra fluid to balance losses in sweat.

GET ENOUGH CALORIES

The number of calories you need depends on your gender, age, height, weight, and activity level. This energy is needed to keep your body warm and functioning normally, to support immune and reproductive functions, to maintain your body tissues, and to keep your muscles moving. Larger individuals need more calories than smaller ones; younger people need more than older ones; men usually need more calories than women do; and more active people need more than less active ones. If you consume fewer calories than you need, fat and lean tissue from the body will be used as fuel, and body weight will decrease. This is good if you are trying to lose weight, but it is not beneficial to athletic performance. To maintain body weight and optimize performance, athletes must be in a state of energy balance. This means that energy intake from food, beverages, and supplements is equal to the energy expended to support body processes, to digest and use food, and to power voluntary physical activity (Figure 4.1).

The amount of energy required for an activity depends on the intensity and duration of that activity. More intense activity requires more energy per unit of time (calories per minute), but the longer an activity continues, the more energy it consumes. Therefore, although weight lifting may require more calories per minute, a distance cyclist usually has higher energy needs than a weight lifter because cyclists continue their activity for longer periods of time.

The DRIs have developed equations to estimate calorie requirements based on individual characteristics and activity levels (see Appendix A). These values are called Estimated Energy Requirements (EERs). Calculating your EER can demonstrate the dramatic impact that activity can have on energy needs. For example, the EER for a 25-year-old, sedentary, 5-foot-11-inch-tall, 70-kg man is 2,510 calories. If this same person becomes a runner and trains several hours per day, his energy needs may increase to 3,510 calories per day or more. Some athletes require as many as 6,000 calories a day to maintain body weight. Table 4.1 illustrates how much energy is needed per hour for various activities.

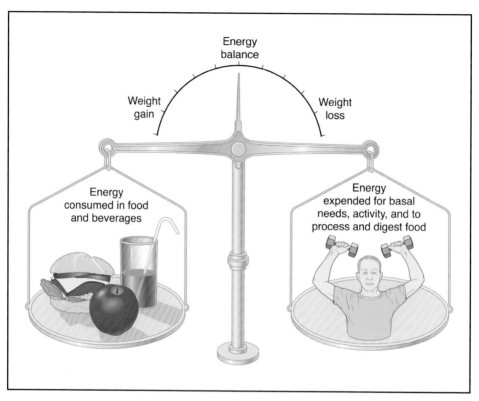

Figure 4.1 When the amount of energy expended by the body is equal to the amount taken in, body weight will remain stable. You can gain or lose weight by adjusting your energy intake, relative to the amount of daily activity in which you take part.

HOW MUCH CARBOHYDRATE, FAT, AND PROTEIN DO ATHLETES NEED?

Carbohydrates, fat, and protein are needed in the proper proportions to maintain fuel production during activity and prevent losses of essential body tissues. Carbohydrates are needed to provide energy and maintain blood glucose levels during exercise. They are also necessary for replacing glycogen stores after exercise. The amount of carbohydrates recommended for athletes depends on their total energy expenditure, the type of sport in which they participate, and the environmental conditions in which they exercise. Generally, needs range from 6 to 10 grams per kilogram of body weight per day.[7] For a 150-pound (68-kg) person burning 3,000 calories per day, this would equal about 60% of calories from carbohydrates. Most of the carbohydrates in the diet should be complex carbohydrates from whole grains and starchy vegetables, with some naturally occurring simple sugars found in fruit and milk. Before or during competition, however, low-fiber snacks are best because they leave the stomach quickly. A full stomach during exercise can cause cramping and GI distress.

Fat is an important source of energy for exercise. It also provides essential fatty acids and is necessary for the absorption of fat-soluble vitamins. Body stores of fat provide enough energy to support the needs of even the longest endurance

---

FACT BOX 4.1

Fueling the Tour de France

What should you eat before you go for a bike ride? How about if your bike ride is 100 to 140 miles (161 to 225 km) a day for three weeks? The Tour de France is just such a ride. Cyclists race around France for three weeks each July, covering over 2,000 miles (3,219 km). The riders travel this distance at an average speed of about 25 miles (40 km) per hour. To provide fuel for this endurance event, they eat an average of 6,000 to 7,000 calories a day and, on some days, need to eat as many as 9,000 to 10,000 calories. Despite this high caloric intake, riders usually lose about 4 to 7 pounds (1.8 to 3.2 kg) over the course of the event. To meet the high calorie demands of this event, athletes use a combination of liquid nutrition and normal meals and snacks. When they are not on their bikes, they eat meals and snack almost continuously, but because they ride for 5 to 6 hours a day, they need to eat while riding as well. To provide for this, team cars follow the riders to supply water, sports drinks, and snacks. Sacks of snacks that the riders can hang around their necks are also passed out at "feeding stations" along the course. Riders try to consume 300 to 400 calories per hour while on their bikes.

Table 4.1. Energy Expended for Activity

ACTIVITY	ENERGY (CAL/HR)						
BODY WEIGHT (LB)	110	125	140	155	170	185	200
Sitting							
Male	73	77	81	85	89	93	97
Female	63	66	69	72	76	79	82
Bowling							
Male	121	128	135	142	148	155	162
Female	105	110	115	121	126	131	136
Aerobics							
Male	455	480	506	531	556	582	607
Female	394	413	433	453	472	492	511
Biking (12 mph)							
Male	380	401	422	443	464	486	507
Female	329	345	361	378	394	410	427
Walking (15 min/mi)							
Male	257	271	285	300	314	328	342
Female	222	233	244	255	266	277	288
Gardening							
Male	303	320	337	354	371	388	405
Female	263	276	289	302	315	328	341
Weight lifting							
Male	340	359	378	397	415	434	453
Female	294	309	323	338	352	367	382
Swimming (laps)							
Male	364	384	405	425	445	465	486
Female	315	331	346	362	378	393	409
Dancing							
Male	364	384	405	425	445	465	486
Female	315	331	346	362	378	393	409
Golf (walking w/bag)							
Male	425	448	472	496	519	543	567
Female	368	386	404	422	441	459	477
Jumping rope							
Male	595	628	661	694	727	760	793
Female	515	540	566	591	617	642	668
Running (10 min/mi)							
Male	619	653	688	722	757	791	826
Female	536	562	589	615	642	669	695

events. For physically active individuals, diets providing 20–25% of energy as fat have been recommended to allow adequate carbohydrate intake and facilitate weight management where necessary.[7] Because fat leaves the stomach slowly, high-fat foods should be avoided before or during exercise to reduce stress on the GI tract.

Protein plays a critical role in the health and performance of athletes. Protein is not a significant energy source, accounting for only about 5% of energy expended, but it is nonetheless needed to maintain and repair lean tissues, including muscle. Eating extra protein, however, does not produce bigger muscles. Muscle growth is stimulated by exercise, not by increasing protein intake. A diet that contains the RDA for protein (0.8 g/kg) provides adequate protein for most active individuals. Competitive athletes who participate in endurance and strength sports may require more protein. In endurance events such as marathons, protein is used for energy and to maintain blood glucose, so athletes who take part in such activities may benefit from 1.2 to 1.4 grams of protein per kilogram per day. Strength athletes who require amino acids to synthesize new muscle proteins may benefit from 1.6 to 1.7 grams per kilogram per day.[7] This amount, however, is not much more than what is contained in the diets of typical American athletes. For example, an 85-kg (187-pound) man who consumes 3,000 calories, 18% of which comes from protein, would be consuming 135 g of protein, or 1.6 g of protein per kg body weight. If the diet is adequate in energy, the recommended amount of dietary protein can easily be consumed without protein or amino acid supplements.

VITAMIN AND MINERAL NEEDS

An adequate supply of each of the vitamins and minerals is crucial to exercise performance. These nutrients are needed for energy production, oxygen delivery, repair and maintenance of body structures, and antioxidant protection.

The B vitamins thiamin, riboflavin, niacin, vitamin B_6, pantothenic acid, and biotin are particularly important for the production of energy from carbohydrates and fats. Vitamin B_6, folate, and vitamin B_{12} are needed for proper synthesis of red blood cells, which deliver oxygen to body tissues. Vitamin B_6 is needed to make the protein hemoglobin, which carries oxygen in red blood cells. Folate and vitamin B_{12} are needed for cell division and, thus, for the synthesis of new red blood cells.

The minerals calcium, iron, and zinc also have important roles in exercise. Calcium is needed to build and repair bones. It is also essential for muscle contraction and the transmission of nerve signals. Iron is important for exercise because it is required for the formation of hemoglobin as well as myoglobin, a protein that increases the amount of oxygen available to the muscle. A number of iron-containing proteins are also needed for production of energy by aerobic metabolism. Zinc is important during exercise because of its role in growth, synthesis, and repair of muscle tissue, as well as energy production. Although these minerals are often low in the diets of athletes, especially female athletes, requirements are no greater than for nonathletes.

Vitamins and minerals with antioxidant function are also important during exercise. Exercise increases the amount of oxygen at the muscle and the rate of chemical reactions that produce energy. These chemical reactions generate dangerous oxygen compounds that can cause oxidative damage to tissues. Antioxidants, such as vitamins C and E; beta-carotene; and selenium protect the body from oxidative damage. Research examining whether exercise increases the need for antioxidant nutrients has so far proven inconclusive.

Exercise has been hypothesized to increase the need for vitamins and minerals because it stresses many metabolic pathways that require these nutrients, it may increase losses from the body, or it may increase the amounts needed for repair and maintenance. Despite this, in most cases, a diet that provides the amounts of vitamins and minerals recommended by the DRIs will still meet the needs of athletes. In addition, because energy needs are increased by activity, a diet that provides enough food to meet the energy needs of an athlete will most likely provide sufficient vitamins and minerals. Therefore, athletes who consume a balanced diet that meets energy needs will also meet their micronutrient needs. Athletes who consume low-fat diets, restrict their intake of energy or specific food groups, or have limited intakes of fruits and vegetables may be at risk for vitamin or mineral deficiencies.

WHAT SHOULD ATHLETES EAT?

The Food Guide Pyramid is a good place to begin when planning an athlete's diet. However, in many cases, an athlete's calorie needs will exceed those provided by the maximum number of servings recommended by the Food Guide Pyramid. In this case, servings should be increased from each of the food groups so that the overall diet still stacks up to be a pyramid with an extra serving or two from each group.

Athletes also need to pay attention to the timing and composition of their meals. Food and fluid intake should be timed around workouts and competitions, and should consider the athlete's individual response to particular foods and meals. Those involved in heavy training may need to eat more than 3 meals and 3 snacks per day to meet calorie needs.

The Pre-exercise Meal: What to Eat Before You Compete

Most of us don't perform at our best when we are hungry. It has been shown that athletes do better after eating a small meal than when exercising in a fasting state. The size, composition, and timing of the pre-exercise meal are important. The wrong meal can hinder performance more than the right one can enhance it.

Ideally, the meal should provide enough fluid to maintain hydration and should be high in carbohydrates (60–70% of calories) to maintain blood glucose and maximize glycogen stores while minimizing hunger and gastric distress. Muscle glycogen is only depleted by exercise, but liver glycogen is used to supply glucose to the blood and is therefore depleted even during rest if no food is ingested. A high-carbohydrate meal, eaten 2 to 4 hours before the event, will fill liver glycogen stores. This meal should also be low in fat (10–25% of calories) and fiber to minimize GI distress, moderate in protein (10–20% of calories), and should consist of foods that are familiar to the athlete. For example, a pancake breakfast or a plate of pasta with marinara sauce would be good choices. Spicy foods, which may cause heartburn, and large amounts of simple sugars, which could cause diarrhea, should also be avoided unless the athlete is accustomed to eating these foods.

In addition to providing nutritional benefits, a meal that includes "lucky" foods may provide some athletes with an added psychological advantage. Because foods affect people differently, athletes should test the effects of these meals and snacks during training, not during competition.

What to Eat on the Run

Fluid consumption is essential during all types of exercise, but for exercise that lasts more than an hour, carbohydrate consumption can also be beneficial. An intake of 0.7 grams of carbohydrates per

---

FACT BOX 4.2

Better Have Breakfast

When you sleep you don't eat, but your heart continues to beat, your lungs expand, and your kidneys filter. All of these processes require energy. This energy is provided by blood glucose derived from the breakdown of liver glycogen. By morning, your liver glycogen stores are only about half what they were the night before. If you start exercising with your glycogen tank half full, you are going to hit empty a lot sooner than you would if you had started with a full tank. Breakfast will fill up your tank. If you plan to exercise at an intense level for more than an hour, you should plan to get up early enough to eat a good breakfast a couple of hours before the activity.

---

kilogram of body weight per hour helps maintain blood glucose and enhance performance. This equates to about 50 grams per hour for a 150-pound (68-kg) person, the equivalent of drinking 3-1/2 cups (0.8 liters) of Gatorade® per hour. For activities that last one hour or less, consuming carbohydrates is unlikely to improve performance. However, it is also not likely to impair performance, and current research supports the consumption of carbohydrates in the amounts typically contained in sports drinks (4–8%). This is particularly important for athletes who exercise in the morning, when liver glycogen levels are low.

Carbohydrate intake should begin shortly after exercise commences and regular amounts should be consumed every 15 to 20 minutes during exercise. The carbohydrates should provide a combination of glucose and fructose. Fructose alone is not very effective and may cause diarrhea. Some athletes may prefer to obtain their carbohydrates from a sports drink, but consuming a solid food snack or a gel with water is also appropriate.

During exercise, sodium and other minerals are lost through sweat. Although the amounts lost during exercise lasting less than 3 to 4 hours are usually not enough to affect health or performance a snack or beverage that contains sodium is recommended for exercise lasting one hour or more. Sodium enhances the palatability of beverages and increases the drive to drink, so even if sodium losses are small, consuming it during exercise may cause an increase in fluid intake.

What to Eat When You're Done: Post-exercise Meals

After exercise, athletes need to replenish fluid, electrolyte, and glycogen losses. When exercise ends, the body must shift from the catabolic state of breaking down glycogen, triglycerides, and muscle proteins for fuel to the anabolic state of restoring muscle and liver glycogen, depositing lipids, and synthesizing muscle proteins. Fluids are essential; choosing a beverage other than plain water can help replace electrolytes. Carbohydrates are needed to replace glycogen stores. Glucose and sucrose are equally effective, but fructose alone is less effective. Protein won't affect glycogen synthesis but will provide amino acids needed for muscle repair.

The first priority for all exercisers is to replace fluid losses. Whether food is needed immediately and what should be eaten depends on the length and intensity of the exercise session and when the next exercise session will occur. If glycogen was not depleted during the event, food may not be needed until the athlete feels hungry. If it was depleted, the time that the next exercise session is scheduled determines how fast it needs to be replenished to ensure maximum performance. When timed properly, post-exercise carbohydrate intake can replenish muscle and liver glycogen stores within 24 hours of the athletic event. The body is most efficient at replenishing carbohydrate stores during the first hour after exercise. Therefore, to maximize glycogen replacement, a high-carbohydrate meal or drink should be consumed as soon as possible after the athletic event and again every 2 hours for 6 hours after the activity. Ideally, the drinks or meals should provide about

---

FACT BOX 4.3

Don't Forget the Fluids!

Many endurance athletes do not like to eat during competition, but consuming carbohydrates is essential if they want to continue high-intensity exercise. To avoid eating solid foods, many athletes have begun to use energy gels as a source of carbohydrates. These high-carbohydrate gels come in a foil packet and can be squeezed into the mouth. Each packet typically contains 25 grams of carbohydrate; consuming 1 to 2 packs per hour will provide sufficient carbohydrates to maintain the body's supplies. These gels are light to carry and provide a low-fiber, high-carbohydrate snack that is easy on the stomach and doesn't cause bloating. However, gels don't provide fluid. Without sufficient fluid, carbohydrate and water absorption are slowed and performance is affected. In order to stay hydrated, athletes need to consume about 2 cups (half a liter) of water with each 25-gram gel pack.

1.5 grams of carbohydrates per kg of body weight, which is about 100 grams of carbohydrate for a 68-kg (150-pound) person—the equivalent of two pancakes with syrup and a glass of fruit punch. This type of regimen to restore glycogen is critical for athletes who have to perform again the next day, but is not necessary if the athlete has one or more days to replace glycogen stores before the next intense exercise session. In the latter case, carbohydrates can be provided over a 24-hour period, and the timing of intake does not affect the amount stored. Approximately 600 grams of carbohydrate, or about 8 to 10 g per kg, should be consumed during the 24 hours after an endurance exercise session that depletes glycogen.

If you typically spend 30 to 60 minutes working out at the gym, you do not need a special glycogen replacement strategy to ensure your stores are full by your next gym visit. A typical diet providing about 55% carbohydrate will replace the glycogen used during your trip to the gym so you will be ready to work out again the next day.

Maximizing Stored Glycogen Can Keep You Going

For the serious endurance athlete, larger muscle glycogen stores allow exercise to continue for longer periods. One way to maximize glycogen stores before an event is to follow a regimen of glycogen supercompensation, or **carbohydrate loading**. This six-day regimen involves depleting glycogen stores with exercise and a diet moderate in carbohydrates, and then replenishing glycogen by consuming a high-carbohydrate diet for a few days before competition, during which time only light exercise is performed. The practice currently suggested is to consume a diet containing about 50% carbohydrate for the first 3 days and then, during the next 3 days, increase this to 70% carbohydrate. Exercise should begin with a 90-minute workout on day 1 and then gradually taper down in duration so that the day before competition—day 6—is a rest day. Increases in glycogen stores occur only in the specific muscles depleted, so it is important to exercise the same muscles that will be used in the event. Because consuming this much carbohydrate can be difficult, there are a number of high-carbohydrate beverages available that contain 50 to 60 grams of carbohydrate in 8 fluid ounces. These should not be confused with sports drinks designed to be consumed during competition, which contain only about 10 to 16 grams of carbohydrate in 8 fluid ounces (0.24 liters). A glycogen supercompensation regimen will increase the amount of muscle glycogen from about 1.7 grams of glycogen per 100 grams to 4 to 5 grams per 100 grams.[8]

Although glycogen supercompensation is beneficial to endurance athletes, it will provide no benefit and even has some disadvantages for those who exercise for periods shorter than 60 minutes. For every gram of glycogen in the muscle, almost 3 grams of water are also deposited. This water will cause a 2- to 7-pound (1- to 3.2-kg) weight gain and may result in some muscle stiffness. As glycogen is used, the water is released. Although this can be an advantage when exercising in hot weather, the extra weight may cancel any potential benefits from increased stores, especially for short-duration events.

CONNECTIONS

Athletes require more fluid and energy than nonathletes do. The proportions of carbohydrates, fat, and protein must be adequate to maintain fuel production during activity and to prevent losses of essential body tissues. Although certain vitamins and minerals have particularly important roles that support exercise, a diet that provides the amounts recommended by the DRIs will still meet an athlete's needs. Because energy needs are increased by activity, a varied diet that is adequate in energy will provide sufficient vitamins and minerals for most individuals. Food eaten before, during, and after competition can affect exercise performance. To maximize energy stores and minimize gastro-intestinal distress during an event, a pre-exercise meal should be consumed 2 to 4 hours before athletic competition. The ideal meal is high in carbohydrates and fluid and low in fat and fiber, which can slow stomach emptying. During exercise, it is impor-tant to replace lost fluids and, for exercise lasting more than an hour, the consumption of carbohydrates and sodium, along with fluid, is recommended. After competition, food and drink should be consumed to replace fluid, electrolyte, and glycogen losses. To load muscle glycogen stores to the maximum, endurance athletes can follow a diet and exercise regime called glycogen supercompensation. This six-day regimen, however, may be a disadvantage for short events.

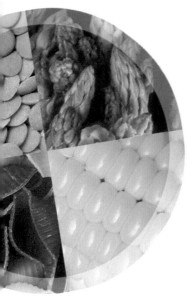

5

Keeping Cool: Water and Electrolyte Balance During Exercise

Your body is made up of about 60% water—this means that water is its most abundant component. You could probably live for 8 weeks without food, but without sufficient water, you would only survive for 3 to 4 days.

Body water contains dissolved substances, including the minerals sodium, potassium, and chloride. These are referred to as **electrolytes** because they are capable of conducting an electrical current when dissolved in water. Electrolytes help regulate the distribution of water throughout the body. Because water cannot be stored, water intake must be balanced with water losses to maintain homeostasis. Exercise increases the loss of water and electrolytes. If not replaced, these losses can impair exercise performance and the desire to perform work.

WHERE IS THE WATER IN YOUR BODY?

Water is found in varying proportions in all the tissues of the body. Some of this water is found inside cells and is known as **intracellular fluid**. Some is located outside of cells and is called **extracellular fluid**. About a third of the water in your body is extracellular fluid. Most of this is fluid between cells, called **interstitial fluid**, and the rest is water in blood plasma, lymph, and cavities, such as that inside the GI tract, eyes, joints, and spinal cord.

Dissolved substances such as sodium, chloride, and potassium (as well as magnesium, calcium, and many other small molecules) play an important role in regulating where water is located in the body. Water can move freely between the different body compartments by osmosis. **Osmosis** is the movement of water across a membrane from an area with a low concentration of dissolved substances to an area with a high concentration of dissolved substances. Therefore, it is the concentrations of dissolved substances that determine the distribution of water among the various compartments. For example, if the concentration of sodium in the blood is high, water from the interstitial fluid is drawn into the blood, diluting the sodium. Electrolytes help maintain fluid balance within the body by helping to keep water within a particular compartment. Electrolyte concentration is also important in regulating the total amount of body water. As a result, adequate water intake and electrolyte balance are both important for proper fluid balance during exercise.

WHAT DOES WATER DO?

Water has many functions in the body. It transports nutrients and other substances; it provides structure and protection; it is needed for numerous chemical reactions; and it is extremely important for the regulation of body temperature.

Water Transports Substances

Water bathes the cells of the body and serves as a transport medium to deliver nutrients to cells and remove wastes. Blood, which is 90% water, transports oxygen, nutrients, hormones, drugs, and other substances to cells. It then carries carbon dioxide and other waste products away from the cells for elimination from the body. During exercise, the need for oxygen and nutrients at the muscle cells increases, as does the production of wastes. Therefore, the need for water as a transport medium is even more crucial during exercise.

Water Provides Structure and Protection

Water is a part of the structure of a number of molecules, including glycogen and proteins. It also makes up most of the volume of body cells. Muscle is about 75% water, and even bone is 25% water. Water helps protect the body by serving as a lubricant and cleanser. Watery tears moisten the eyes and wash away dirt, synovial fluid lubricates the joints, and saliva keeps the mouth moist, making it easier to chew and swallow food. Water also protects the body by acting as a cushion. For example, fluids inside the eyeballs and spinal cord act as cushions against shock.

Water Is Needed for Chemical Reactions

Water is involved in numerous chemical reactions throughout the body. It serves as the medium in which all metabolic reactions occur. Water is an ideal solvent because the two ends of the water molecule have different electrical charges—one end is positive and one end is negative. This property allows water to surround other charged molecules and disperse them. For example, table salt consists of a positively charged sodium ion and a negatively charged chloride ion. When placed in water, the sodium and chloride ions move apart because the positively charged sodium ion is attracted to the negative end of the water molecule and the negatively charged chloride ion is attracted to the positive end.

Water also participates directly in a number of chemical reactions, many of which are involved in energy production. The addition of water to a large molecule can break it into two smaller ones. Likewise, the removal of a water molecule can join two molecules together. Some of the reactions in which water participates help maintain the proper level of acidity in the body. Acid balance in the body is regulated by chemical reactions in body fluids, gas exchange in the lungs, and filtration in the kidneys. Water plays an important role in each of these. Acid balance is particularly important during exercise when lactic acid is formed. The ability to eliminate this acid prevents changes in blood and muscle acidity and is essential for exercise to continue.

Water Regulates Body Temperature

Exercise generates heat. This occurs because the efficiency of converting the chemical energy in ATP into the mechanical energy of muscle contraction is only about 20–25%. The excess energy (the other 75–80%) is lost as heat. In addition, the aerobic and anaerobic metabolic reactions needed to produce ATP generate heat. For exercise to continue, the body must dissipate this heat. Water plays a crucial role in eliminating heat during exercise.

The water in blood helps regulate body temperature by increasing or decreasing the amount of heat lost at the body surface. When body temperature starts to rise, the blood vessels in the skin dilate, causing blood to flow close to the surface of the body, where it can release some of the heat into the environment. This is the reason your skin reddens in hot weather or during strenuous activity. In a cold environment, the opposite occurs. The blood vessels in the skin constrict, restricting the flow of blood near the surface and conserving body heat.

The most obvious way that water helps regulate body temperature is through the evaporation of sweat. When body temperature increases, the brain triggers the sweat glands in the skin to produce sweat, which is mostly water. As the sweat evaporates from the skin, heat is lost, cooling the body.

WATER INTAKE

Water in the body comes from water in the diet—mostly as water itself and other fluids, but also from solid food. For example, low-fat milk is 90% water, apples are about 85% water, and meat is about 50% water (Figure 5.1). A small amount of water is generated inside the body through metabolism, but this is not significant in meeting the body's water needs.

Water is absorbed from the gastrointestinal tract by osmosis. The volume of water and the density of nutrients consumed with it influence the rate of absorption. Consuming a large volume of water increases its rate of absorption. Water consumed alone will easily move from the intestine into the blood, where the concentration of solutes (dissolved substances) is higher. When water is consumed with meals, absorption is slower because the concentration of dissolved substances in the intestine is higher. As the nutrients from the meal move from the intestine into the plasma, the solute concentration in the intestine decreases and water moves by osmosis toward the area with the highest solute concentration.

About 1.7 liters of water enter the GI tract each day from the diet. Another 7 liters come from saliva and other gastrointestinal secretions. Most of this fluid is absorbed in the small intestine but a small amount is also absorbed in the colon.

Balancing Water Intake and Losses

To maintain water homeostasis, intake and excretion must balance. Water intake is stimulated by thirst but is not precisely regulated. Water loss by the kidneys is regulated more precisely by adjusting urinary losses. Electrolytes are lost in urine and sweat. The kidney regulates the amounts lost in urine over a wide range of intakes, making electrolyte imbalances unlikely in healthy people. The amounts lost in sweat are small but if the volume of sweat lost is great, these losses, particularly the loss of sodium, can add up and affect health.

Thirst

How do you know when you need water? The need to consume water or other fluids is signaled by the sensation of thirst. Thirst is triggered both by sensations in the mouth and signals from the brain.

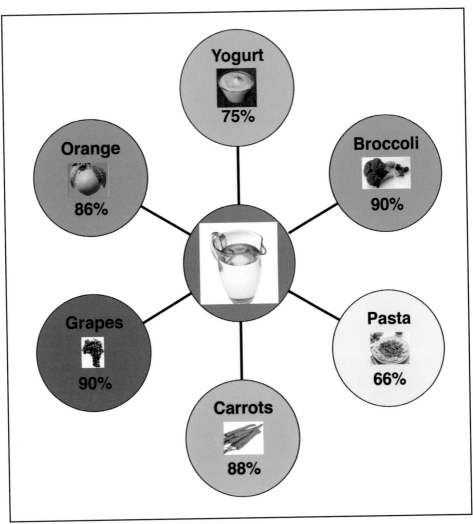

Figure 5.1 Water is consumed in fluids but many foods are also good sources of water. The percentages in each circle indicate the amount of that food's weight that comes from water.

The mouth becomes dry because less water is available for saliva. The thirst center in the brain senses a decrease in the amount of fluid in blood and an increase in the concentration of dissolved substances in this fluid. Together, the feeling of a dry mouth and signals from the brain cause the sensation of thirst and motivate us to drink.

Thirst is not a perfect regulator of water intake. It is quenched almost as soon as fluid is consumed and long before water balance has been restored. Also, the sensation of thirst often lags behind the actual need for water. For example, athletes exercising in hot weather lose water rapidly but do not experience intense thirst until they have lost so much body water that their physical performance is compromised.[9] Also, being thirsty does not mean that you will take a drink. Because people cannot and do not always respond to thirst, water loss from the body is regulated by the kidneys to prevent **dehydration**.

Water and Electrolyte Losses

Water is removed from the body in urine, feces, and through evaporation from the lungs and skin. A typical young man loses about 2.75 liters of water daily.

Average urine output is about 1 to 2 liters per day, but this varies depending on the amount of fluid consumed and the amount of waste to be excreted. The waste products that must be excreted in urine include **urea** and other nitrogen-containing products from protein breakdown, **ketones** from fat breakdown, phosphates, sulfates, electrolytes, and other minerals. The amount of urea that must be excreted increases when dietary protein intake or body protein breakdown rises. Ketone excretion is increased when body fat is broken down, such as during weight loss. The amount of sodium that must be excreted goes up when more is consumed in the diet. In all of these cases, the need for water increases in order to produce more urine to excrete the extra wastes.

The amount of water lost in the feces is usually small, only about 100 to 200 ml per day (less than a cup). This is remarkable, because every day about 9 liters of fluid enter the gastrointestinal tract via food, water, and gastrointestinal secretions. Under normal conditions, more than 95% of this fluid is reabsorbed before the feces are eliminated. However, in cases of severe diarrhea, large amounts of water can be lost through the gastrointestinal tract.

Water loss due to evaporation from the skin and respiratory tract takes place continuously. These losses are referred to as

insensible losses because the individual is unaware that they are occurring. An inactive person at room temperature loses about 1,000 ml per day through insensible losses, but the amount varies depending on body size, environmental temperature and humidity, and physical activity. For example, more water is lost when the humidity is low, such as in the desert, than it would be on a rainy day.

Water is also lost in sweat. The amount of water lost via sweat is extremely variable depending on environmental conditions (temperature, humidity, wind speed, radiant heat), clothing, exercise intensity, level of physical training, and the degree to which the exerciser is acclimatized to his or her environment. Sweat rate increases as exercise intensity builds and as the environment becomes hotter and more humid. An individual doing light work at a temperature of about 84°F (29°C) will lose about 2–3 liters of sweat per day. Strenuous exercise in a hot environment can cause water losses in sweat to be as high as 2–4 liters in an hour.[10] Clothing that allows sweat to evaporate will help the body cool and will decrease sweat losses. Athletes who are more highly trained as well as those accustomed to a hot environment tend to sweat more.

A cold environment can also increase the amount of water lost from the body. Cold air is less humid, so more water is lost through evaporation from the respiratory tract. Cold stress also stimulates an increase in urine production and, therefore, in water losses. Dissipating the heat produced while exercising in a cold environment can be difficult because of clothing. People often overdress, so as exercise proceeds, the excess heat produced cannot be let out into the environment.

Altitude is another factor that may increase water loss from the body. Altitudes higher than 8,200 feet (2,500 meters) increase urinary losses and evaporative respiratory losses, and decrease appetite. The increase in urine output lasts for about 7 days and increases water loss by about 500 ml per day. Due to the dry air at high altitudes, respiratory water losses may be as high as 1,900 ml per day in men and 850 ml per day in women. The decrease in appetite reduces voluntary fluid intake. Fluid intake per day at high altitude should be increased to as much as 3–4 liters per day.

Kidneys Regulate Water and Electrolyte Excretion

The kidneys serve as a filtering system that regulates the amount of water and dissolved substances retained in the blood and excreted in urine. As blood flows through the kidneys, water and small molecules are filtered out of the blood vessels. Some of the water and molecules are reabsorbed and the rest are excreted in the urine. The amount of water and electrolytes that are reabsorbed depends on conditions in the body. There are two hormonal systems that regulate fluid and electrolyte balance.

One system that regulates water balance detects changes in the concentration of solutes in the blood. When the concentration is high, the pituitary gland secretes **antidiuretic hormone (ADH)**. This hormone signals the kidneys to reabsorb water, reducing the amount lost in the urine. The reabsorbed water is then returned to the blood, decreasing the solute concentration to normal. When the solute concentration in the blood is low, ADH levels decrease, so less water is reabsorbed and more is excreted in the urine, allowing blood solute concentration to increase to normal.

The other system that regulates the amount of water in the body is activated by changes in blood pressure and relies on the ability of the kidneys to conserve sodium. Because water follows sodium by osmosis, changes in the amount of sodium retained or excreted result in changes in the amount of body water. Sodium is the primary determinant of extracellular fluid volume. When the concentration of sodium in the blood decreases, water moves out of the blood, causing a decrease in blood volume. A decrease in blood volume causes a decrease in blood pressure. When blood pressure decreases, the kidneys release the enzyme **renin**, beginning a series of events leading to the production of **angiotensin II** (Figure 5.2). Angiotensin II increases blood pressure both by causing the blood vessel walls to constrict and by stimulating the release of the hormone **aldosterone**, which acts on the kidneys to increase sodium reabsorption. Water follows the reabsorbed sodium, and is returned to the blood. As blood pressure returns to normal, it inhibits the release of renin and aldosterone so that blood pressure does not continue to rise.

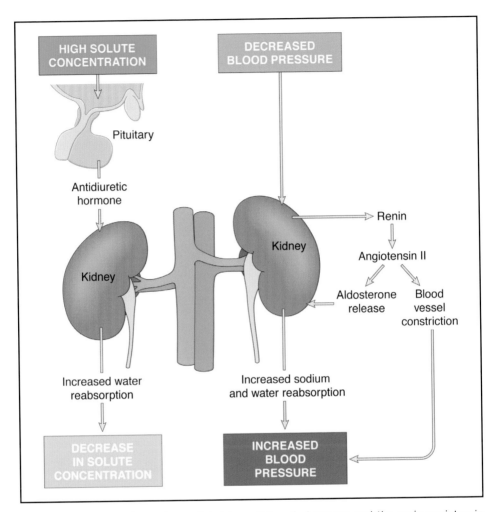

Figure 5.2 Fluid balance is regulated by antidiuretic hormone and the renin-angiotensin system, which triggers the release of the hormone aldosterone. When the body senses changes in its overall water level, it uses these systems to keep its fluids in balance.

The kidneys also regulate chloride and potassium excretion to maintain relatively constant amounts in the body. In the case of potassium, a rise in blood levels stimulates cellular uptake of potassium. This short-term regulation prevents the amount of potassium in the extracellular fluid from rising to lethal levels. The long-term regulation of potassium balance, like that of sodium, depends on aldosterone release, which causes the kidney to excrete potassium and retain sodium.

PROBLEMS WITH FLUID AND ELECTROLYTE BALANCE

During exercise, most people only drink enough to assuage their thirst. As a result, they end their exercise session in a state of dehydration and must restore fluid balance during the post-exercise period. Even when endurance athletes consume fluids at regular intervals throughout exercise, they often cannot take in enough to compensate for losses from sweat and evaporation through the lungs. Dehydration hastens the onset of fatigue and makes exercise seem more difficult.

Dehydration

Dehydration results when water losses exceed water intake. Dehydration severe enough to cause clinical symptoms can occur more rapidly than any other nutrient deficiency. Likewise, health can be restored in a matter of minutes or hours if fluid is replaced.

Early symptoms of dehydration include headache, fatigue, loss of appetite, dry eyes and mouth, and dark-colored urine. Even mild dehydration—a body water loss of 1% to about 2% of body weight—can impair physical and cognitive performance.[11] A 3% reduction in body weight can significantly reduce cardiac output because an increase in heart rate cannot compensate for the reduction in stroke volume. This decreases the ability of the circulatory system to deliver oxygen and nutrients to cells and remove waste products. The lowered blood volume that occurs with dehydration reduces blood flow to the skin and sweat production, which limits the body's ability to sweat and cool itself. Core body temperature can then increase and, with it, the risk of various heat-related illnesses. As water losses increase, a proportionately greater percentage of the water is lost from intracellular spaces. This water is needed to maintain metabolic functions. A loss of 5% body weight as water can cause nausea and difficulty concentrating. When water loss approaches 7% of body weight, confusion and disorientation may occur. A loss of about 10 to 20% can result in death (Figure 5.3).

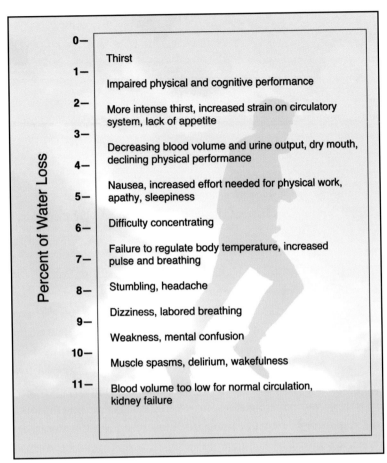

Percent of Water Loss

0—
1— Thirst

Impaired physical and cognitive performance

2— More intense thirst, increased strain on circulatory system, lack of appetite

3—

Decreasing blood volume and urine output, dry mouth, declining physical performance

4—

Nausea, increased effort needed for physical work, apathy, sleepiness

5—

Difficulty concentrating

6—

Failure to regulate body temperature, increased pulse and breathing

7—

Stumbling, headache

8—

Dizziness, labored breathing

9—

Weakness, mental confusion

10—

Muscle spasms, delirium, wakefulness

11—

Blood volume too low for normal circulation, kidney failure

Figure 5.3 As the percentage of water loss increases, the effects of dehydration become more severe. If fluid is not restored quickly, dehydration can ultimately lead to death.

Low Sodium: Hyponatremia

Sweat is important for cooling the body. Sweat is mostly water and, for most activities, sweat losses can be replaced with ordinary water. However, sweat also contains some minerals, primarily sodium and chloride with smaller amounts of potassium, and during prolonged exercise, the loss of sodium through sweat can be great enough to affect health and performance. A reduction in the level of sodium in the blood is referred to as **hyponatremia**. This condition can occur if an athlete loses large amounts of water and salt in sweat, then tries to replace the loss with water alone. This causes the sodium that remains in blood to be diluted, making the amount of water too great for the amount of sodium. This might be compared to taking a full glass of salt water, dumping out half, and replacing what was poured out with plain water. The sodium in the glass is now diluted. Athletes can lose 2–3 grams of salt per liter of sweat. It is not unusual for an athlete to lose a liter of sweat per hour, so he or she may sweat away 20 or more grams of salt during a 10-hour competition. It is also possible to develop hyponatremia even when salt losses from sweating are not excessive. This can occur if an athlete drinks too much water, which dilutes the sodium in the system. For example, an athlete may overhydrate while exercising in a cooler climate in which sweat losses are lower. It is the concentration of sodium that is important, not the absolute amount.

Hyponatremia causes a number of problems. Solutes in the blood help hold fluid in the blood vessels. As sodium concentration drops, fluid will leave the bloodstream by osmosis and accumulate in the tissues, causing swelling. Fluid accumulation in the lungs inter-feres with gas exchange, and fluid accumulation in the brain causes disorientation, seizure, coma, and even death. The early symptoms of hyponatremia may be similar to those of dehydration: nausea, muscle cramps, disorientation, slurred speech, and confusion. Drink-ing water alone will make the problem worse and can result in seizure, coma, or death.

Hyponatremia is a serious concern in endurance events that take place in hot environments. It is estimated that approximately 30% of the finishers of the Hawaii Iron Man competition are both hyponatremic and dehydrated.[12] Mild symptoms of hyponatremia can be treated by eating salty foods or drinking a sodium-containing beverage such as a sports drink. More severe symptoms require medical attention. Hyponatremia can be prevented by using sodium-containing sports drinks during long-distance events, increasing sodium intake several days prior to competition, and avoiding Tylenol®, aspirin, ibuprofen, and other nonsteroidal anti-inflammatory agents. These medications interfere with kidney function and may contribute to the development of hyponatremia. Although imbalances of electrolytes can be life-threatening, the replacement of lost water during exercise is usually far more of a concern than the replacement of lost electrolytes. For most types of exercise, lost electrolytes can be replaced during the meals following exercise.

Heat-Related Illness

During exercise, heat production increases along with exercise intensity. If heat cannot be emitted from the body, then body temperature rises and exercise performance as well as health may be jeopardized. The ability to dissipate the heat generated during exercise is affected by the hydration status and conditioning of the exerciser as well as by environmental conditions. Dehydration dramatically increases the risk of heat-related illness; conditioning with repeated bouts of exercise can reduce the risks. The effects of environmental conditions depend on both temperature and humidity. As environmental temperature rises, it becomes more difficult for the body to dissipate heat and, as humidity rises, the ability to cool the body by evaporation is lowered. **Apparent temperature** or **heat index** is a measure of how hot it feels

---

FACT BOX 5.1

Hyponatremia Makes Headlines

In the 2002 Boston Marathon, Cynthia Lucero was looking good when she reached the bottom of Heartbreak Hill, just 6 miles (9.65 km) from the finish line. Soon after, at mile 22 (kilometer 35), she collapsed in a coma from which she never recovered. What killed her was a swelling in the brain that resulted from an imbalance of water and sodium. Before her death, most people didn't know that you could drink too much water. In fact, deaths from this condition are extremely rare, but the problem may not be. In a study that examined 18,000 marathon runners, 9% of those who sought medical attention had hyponatremia (low sodium levels in the blood). Because of Lucero's death, athletes and physicians are now aware that both dehydration and hyponatremia are potential problems for endurance athletes.

when the relative humidity is added to the actual temperature. For example, when the humidity is 100%, a temperature of 82°F (28°C) feels the same as a temperature of 90°F (32°C) and a humidity of only 40%. The risks associated with exercising under these conditions are similar.

Dehydration and disturbances in electrolyte balance can result in various types of heat-related illness. These include heat cramps, heat exhaustion, and heat stroke. Heat cramps are involuntary muscle spasms that occur during or after intense exercise, most often in the muscles that were used. They are caused by an imbalance of the electrolytes sodium and potassium at the muscle cell membranes and can occur when water and salt are lost during extended athletic activity.

FACT BOX 5.2

Andersen-Scheiss Demonstrates Dehydration to the World

Gabriele Andersen-Scheiss, a marathoner in the 1984 Olympics, demonstrated to the world the effects of dehydration. When this 37-year-old runner entered the Olympic stadium for her final lap of the women's marathon, she was staggering as if she were drunk. Her left arm hung limp at her side and her right leg was stiff. It wasn't clear whether she could negotiate the final lap around the track to complete the marathon. Medical officers rushed over to help her, but she waved them off. By carefully observing her condition, doctors made the decision to allow her to continue unaided. The physicians could see that although she was seriously dehydrated, she was still sweating. This suggested that she was not yet suffering from heat stroke, the most severe and life-threatening form of heat-related illness. Her final lap around the track to the finish line took 5 minutes and 44 seconds. Medics immediately treated her for heat exhaustion. She recovered rapidly and was released from the hospital after only two hours to return to the Olympic village for dinner. Her struggle to finish allowed her to place 37th in the first women's Olympic marathon. It also demonstrated that dehydration can come on rapidly and have devastating effects, but it can be alleviated faster than any other nutrient deficiency.

Heat exhaustion occurs when fluid loss causes blood volume to decrease so much that it is not possible both to cool the body and deliver oxygen to active muscles. It is characterized by a rapid, weak pulse; low blood pressure; fainting; profuse sweating; and disorientation. Someone experiencing heat exhaustion symptoms should stop exercising immediately and move to a cooler environment. If exercise continues, heat exhaustion may progress to heat stroke.

Heat stroke, the most serious form of heat-related illness, occurs when the temperature regulatory center of the brain fails due to a very high core body temperature (greater than 105°F). Heat stroke is characterized by elevated body temperature; hot, dry skin; extreme confusion; and unconsciousness. It requires immediate medical attention.

Children Are at Risk

Children have a larger surface-to-volume ratio than adults do, which allows them to dissipate heat from the skin more efficiently. Even with this advantage, they are at a greater risk than adults are for heat-related illness because they produce more heat, are less able to transfer heat from muscles to the skin, and sweat less than adults do. To reduce risks, children should rest periodically in the shade, consume fluids frequently, and limit the intensity and duration of activities on hot days. Younger people may also take longer to acclimate to heat, so they should exercise at a reduced intensity and take more time to get used to their conditions than adult competitors would need.

FLUID AND ELECTROLYTE NEEDS

Under average nonexercising conditions, adult men need about 3.7 liters of water per day and women about 2.7 liters per day.[11] This does not all need to be consumed as water; other fluids such as juice, milk, and lemonade can also meet needs. Water and other beverages account for about 80% of adult fluid intake. The other 20% comes from water in foods. Beverages that contain caffeine or alcohol, such as coffee, tea, caffeinated soda, beer, and wine, provide fluid, but they also act as diuretics—which actually increase water loss in the urine. In general, these only increase water loss for

Table 5.1 Recommended Fluid Intake for Exercise

Before Exercise

- Begin exercise well hydrated by consuming generous amounts of fluid in the 24 hours before exercise.
- Consume about half a liter of fluid 2 hours before exercise.

During Exercise

- Consume at least 6 to 12 ounces (0.17 to 0.35 liters) of fluid every 15 to 20 minutes.
- For exercise lasting 60 minutes or less, water is adequate for fluid replacement.
- For exercise lasting longer than 60 minutes, a fluid containing carbohydrates and electrolytes may improve endurance and protect health.

After Exercise

- Begin fluid replacement immediately after exercise.
- Consume 24 ounces (0.71 liters) of fluid for each pound (0.45 kg) of weight lost.

a short period, so they do contribute to fluid needs over the course of the day. However, because of the immediate effect they have on fluid balance, they are not a good beverage choice during exercise (Table 5.1).

Anyone who is exercising should consume extra fluids. Failure to take in adequate fluids to replace water lost through the lungs and in sweat can be critical to even the most casual athlete. For most people who exercise, water is the only fluid needed, but sports drinks have no disadvantages and may offer some benefits. How a beverage affects fluid balance depends on the composition of the beverage consumed, the rate at which it is ingested, how quickly it leaves the stomach, and how fast it is absorbed from the intestines.

A good sports drink should empty from the stomach rapidly, enhance intestinal absorption, and promote fluid retention. To ensure hydration, adequate fluids should be consumed before, during, and after exercise.

What and How Much Should You Drink Before Exercise?

Because water helps cool the body, the risk of heat-related illness is greatly increased when someone begins exercise in a dehydrated condition. Athletes should therefore be well hydrated when they start to exercise. To ensure adequate hydration, exercisers should drink generous amounts of fluid during the 24 hours before the exercise session and about 2 cups (half a liter) of fluid 2 to 3 hours before exercise.

What and How Much Should You Drink During Exercise?

During exercise, whether casual or competitive, exercisers should try to drink enough water to balance water losses. Since thirst is not a reliable indicator of fluid needs, it is important for anyone exercising to schedule fluid breaks. Even with regular fluid intake, however, maintaining fluid balance may not be possible, because sweat rates can exceed the maximal rate at which water empties from the stomach and can be absorbed from the gastrointestinal tract. In most cases, however, the amount of fluid ingested by the athlete does not exceed the amount that can be emptied from the stomach and is not enough to balance fluid losses. Hydration can be optimized by drinking 6 to 12 ounces (0.17 to 0.35 liters) of fluid every 15 to 20 minutes, beginning at the start of exercise. [7]

Intense exercise lasting longer than 60 minutes may cause body carbohydrate stores to be depleted. A beverage containing 4–8 grams of carbohydrate per 100 ml of fluid is therefore recommended. This is the amount of carbohydrate found in popular sports beverages such as Gatorade® and Powerade®. Although not necessary, these beverages are also suitable for exercise lasting less than an hour. The carbohydrates in a beverage help maintain blood glucose levels, thereby providing a source of glucose for the muscles and delaying fatigue. As the amount of carbohydrates in the beverage increases, the rate at which the solution leaves the stomach decreases. Therefore, beverages containing larger amounts of carbohydrates, such as fruit juices and soft drinks, are not recommended unless they are diluted with an equal volume of water. Water and carbohydrate trapped in the stomach do not benefit the athlete.

Sodium and other minerals are lost in sweat. However, the amounts lost during exercise lasting less than 3–4 hours are usually not enough to affect health or performance. Consuming a beverage containing 0.5–0.7 grams of sodium per liter (1.2–1.8 g of sodium chloride per liter) is recommended for exercise lasting one hour or more. This is because the sodium enhances palatability and the drive to drink, so it may encourage the athlete to increase fluid intake. This amount of sodium is greater than the 450 milligrams of sodium per liter found in commercial sports beverages. A sodium-containing beverage will help prevent hyponatremia in athletes who overhydrate and in those participating in endurance events, such as ultramarathons or Iron Man triathlons, when significant amounts of sodium may be lost in sweat.

What and How Much Should You Drink After Exercise?

Typically, exercising individuals ingest amounts of fluids that are equal to only about one- to two-thirds of the amount lost in sweat.[13] They therefore complete their exercise sessions in a state of dehydration. To restore water lost through sweat and urine, about 24 ounces (0.7 liters) of fluid should be consumed for each pound of weight lost

---

FACT BOX 5.3

Make Your Own Sports Drink

Sports drinks really just consist of water, sugar, and salt. You can save some money by making your own. Mix together 4 teaspoons of sugar, 1/4 teaspoon of salt, 8 ounces of water, and some flavoring, such as a teaspoon of lemon juice.

during an exercise session. Consuming a sodium-containing beverage or drinking water along with a sodium-containing food will cause less water to be lost in urine after exercise than would be lost if plain water were consumed. Including sodium will also help maintain the proper concentration of sodium in the blood, and, therefore, the desire to drink. An athlete who has gained weight during an event has consumed more fluid than was lost and is at risk for hyponatremia.

CONNECTIONS

Water is essential for survival. In the body, water transports nutrients and other substances, provides structure and protection, is needed for numerous chemical reactions, and is extremely important in the regulation of body temperature. It is distributed between intracellular and extracellular compartments and moves between these by osmosis. Water cannot be stored, so intake must equal output to maintain hydration. Water is consumed in beverages and food, and small amounts are produced in the body by metabolism. Water is excreted in urine and feces and is lost in sweat and through evaporation from the skin and lungs. Water balance is regulated primarily by the kidney. If body water is low, antidiuretic hormone causes a reduction in urine output and other hormones cause the kidney to retain sodium, thereby increasing water retention. A reduction in body water can have dire consequences for health. Mild dehydration can result in headache, fatigue, loss of appetite, and dark urine. More severe dehydration can affect the functioning of the circulatory system and the body's ability to cool itself. This condition can be fatal. Dehydration can also precipitate other heat-related illnesses, such as heat stress, heat exhaustion, and heat stroke. To prevent these problems, athletes should begin an exercise session well hydrated. During exercise, athletes should try to drink enough fluid to replace losses. For exercise lasting more than an hour, fluids containing sugar and electrolytes are recommended. During prolonged exercise, replacement of fluids with plain water can dilute blood sodium and cause hyponatremia. After exercise, fluid losses can be replaced by drinking 24 ounces (0.7 liters) for every pound of weight lost.

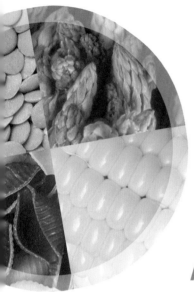

6

Ergogenic Aids for Athletes: Are They Safe?

For as long as there have been athletic competitions, athletes have longed for and experimented with anything that might give them a competitive edge. Everything from desiccated liver to shark's cartilage has been used to enhance athletic performance. Most of these so-called ergogenic aids provide more of a psychological than a physiological edge; some can enhance performance in certain types of activities, but others can actually impair health and prevent an athlete from reaching his or her maximal level of performance.

Anything designed to enhance performance can be considered an ergogenic aid. Running shoes are mechanical aids; psychotherapy is a psychological aid; drugs are pharmacological aids. Special diets and dietary supplements are also used as ergogenic aids. Although many of these supplements are expensive and most have not been shown to improve performance, the thrill of competition and the desire to be the very best may cause athletes to ignore the potential hazards of a supplement and believe the unbelievable.

WEIGHING THE RISKS AND BENEFITS

If you are considering using an ergogenic supplement, it is important to weigh the health risks against potential benefits. Just because a product is sold doesn't make it safe, and just because something appears in print does not mean it is true. The Food and Drug Administration (FDA) does not have the authority to regulate the safety or effectiveness of dietary supplements before they are sold on the market. The agency does regulate the information that appears on supplement labels, but information in magazines, brochures, and advertisements about nutritional ergogenic aids is not regulated and may be inaccurate. Choosing to use an ergogenic aid is a serious decision. The ability to identify products that may be beneficial as opposed to those that are worthless or even harmful is an important skill. Before taking a product, discuss it with your doctor. Many supplements can have dangerous interactions with other medications and may exacerbate existing health conditions. You should also consider whether the claims made about the product are valid, whether the dose recommended is safe, and whether it is ethical to take the substance.

Are the Product Claims Valid?

To determine if claims made about a product are reliable, look beyond the marketing materials. Don't trust one source of information. Look for more articles or the opinion of experts in the

---

FACT BOX 6.1

Who Checks Supplements for Safety?

According to the Dietary Supplement Health and Education Act of 1994, supplement manufacturers are responsible for ensuring that the products they make are safe. The Food and Drug Administration (FDA) is only involved after the product is already on the market. The FDA collects information about suspected problems with dietary supplements and has the authority to remove products from the market if it can prove that a particular product carries significant risk.

---

field of nutrition or exercise. When evaluating a product claim, consider whether the claim makes sense. If it sounds too good to be true, it probably is. For example, products that claim to bring about quick improvements, such as an increase in muscle strength by your next workout, should be viewed skeptically. Products that claim to contain a secret ingredient or formula are also suspicious. Real scientific information and medical advances are published, shared, and scrutinized—they would not be kept secret. Another clue that a product may not be all that it promises is the use of popular TV personalities or star athletes as spokespersons in advertisements. This strategy encourages people to believe that if they use the product, they will look or perform like the spokesperson. The person who promotes a product has no impact on how effective or safe it is.

Consider where the claim about the product came from. Is it from an article in a scientific journal? Is it in a magazine, newspaper, or book? Is it from a company selling a product? Research studies published in reputable scientific journals are the most reliable source of information. Be aware, however, that one research study is never final proof. Several methodologically sound studies are needed to support a theory, and concluding such studies may take years. However, the results of a new study may look too good to wait for this proof and an article in a magazine or newspaper may be based on a single new scientific study. This is not to say that articles in magazines and newspapers are not reliable. They often are, but they are also there to sell magazines. Claims may be exaggerated to make a magazine cover or newspaper headline more appealing to buyers.

Looking at the credentials of the person who wrote the article can also help judge its reliability. Articles written by people with nutrition or sports medicine degrees from accredited colleges or universities or a title such as registered dietitian (RD) are usually reliable.

Is the Product Safe at the Recommended Dose?

Many nutritional supplements are safe at low doses but have adverse effects at high doses. The dose recommended for ergogenic benefits may have side effects that outweigh any benefits. For example, large amounts of caffeine have an ergogenic effect, but in many people, this dose causes intestinal cramps that impair performance. The length of time over which the product must be taken should also be considered. Some ergogenic aids must be used continuously to have an effect, but may be unsafe in the long run. Others are so new that no one knows yet what the long-term effects will be.

Is Taking the Supplement Ethical?

The ancient Greek ideal and the ideal of the International Olympic Committee is that an athlete should triumph through his or her own unaided effort. Everyone must assess his or her own ethical standards, but you should also take into consideration the policy of your team, whether the substance is banned from use during competition, and whether taking it is cheating or giving you an unfair advantage.

ARE VITAMIN SUPPLEMENTS ERGOGENIC?

Do you think vitamins give you energy? They actually don't provide any energy, although they are needed for you to produce energy, and this function as well as others are the reasons many different vitamin supplements are marketed to athletes as ergogenic aids. For example, thiamin, riboflavin, niacin, and pantothenic acid are all involved in muscle energy metabolism. Thiamin and pantothenic acid are needed for carbohydrates to enter the citric acid cycle for aerobic metabolism. Riboflavin and niacin are needed to shuttle electrons to the electron transport chain so ATP can be formed. Vitamin B_6 is needed to use amino acids for energy, to break down muscle glycogen, and to convert lactic acid to glucose in the liver. Vitamins B_6, B_{12}, and folic acid are needed to transport of oxygen to exercising muscle—vitamin B_6 because it is needed for the synthesis of hemoglobin, and folic acid and vitamin B_{12} because they are both involved in the replication of red blood cells. Although a deficiency of one or more of these vitamins would interfere with energy production and impair athletic performance, consuming more than the recommended amounts has not been shown to enhance performance.

The claims that athletes should consume supplements of vitamin E, vitamin C, and beta-carotene focus on their antioxidant functions. Exercise increases oxygen use and oxidative processes. It therefore increases the production of free radicals. Free radicals are reactive chemical substances that can damage tissues and have been associated with fatigue during exercise.[14] It has been suggested that antioxidant supplements prevent free radical damage and delay fatigue, but research examining the effect of exercise on the need for antioxidants has not been conclusive.[7]

Although vitamin supplements may not give an athlete the winning edge, as long as they are not consumed in amounts that exceed the Tolerable Upper Intake Levels (ULs) recommended by the DRIs, there is little risk associated with their use (Appendix B).

ARE MINERAL SUPPLEMENTS ERGOGENIC?

Minerals like chromium and iron sound as tough as nails and many are advertised as being able to make you stronger and faster. Some of the minerals promoted as endurance enhancers include chromium, vanadium, selenium, zinc, and iron. As with vitamin supplements, many of the claims made about these minerals are based on their physiological functions.

Chromium supplements, in the **chromium picolinate** form, claim to increase lean body mass and decrease body fat. Chromium is needed for the hormone insulin to function optimally. One of the actions of insulin is to promote protein synthesis. Therefore, adequate chromium status is likely to be important for lean tissue synthesis. The picolinate form is favored because it is believed to be absorbed better than other forms of chromium. Studies in humans have not consistently demonstrated an effect of supplemental chromium picolinate on muscle strength, body composition, body weight, or other aspects of health.[15] A UL has not been established for chromium, but there is evidence that this supplement may cause DNA damage.[16] This evidence comes from studies done in cells grown in the laboratory. Human studies using the standard supplemental dose of chromium picolinate have not detected an increase in DNA damage, but more work is needed to completely rule out any risk.[17]

Vanadium, usually sold in the form of vanadyl sulfate, is another mineral marketed for its ability to assist the action of insulin. Vanadium supplements promise to increase lean body mass, but there is no evidence that they have a muscle building effect, and toxicity is a concern.[18] A UL of 1.8 mg per day of elemental vanadium has been set for adults age 19 and older.

Selenium is marketed for its antioxidant properties and zinc for its role in protein synthesis and tissue repair, but neither of these supplements has been found to improve athletic performance in individuals with adequate mineral status. Iron is also marketed as an ergogenic mineral because it is needed for hemoglobin synthesis. If an iron deficiency exists, as it frequently does in female athletes, supplements can be of benefit.

DO PROTEIN SUPPLEMENTS STIMULATE MUSCLE GROWTH?

There are hundreds of protein powders and bars available and they are typically marketed with the promise that they will increase muscle size and strength and decrease recovery time. Muscle growth does require additional protein, but, unfortunately, the protein you eat doesn't automatically deposit in your muscles. Muscle growth occurs in response to exercise in the presence of adequate protein. The protein provided by expensive supplements will not meet an athlete's needs any better than the protein found in a balanced diet. The amount of protein needed by athletes is easily obtained from the diet.

Protein supplements are not harmful for most people, but they are an expensive and unnecessary way to increase protein intake. Protein is needed for proper immune function, healthy hair, and muscle growth, but a protein supplement will improve these parameters only if the diet is deficient in protein in the first place. Increasing protein intake above the requirement does not protect you from disease, make your hair shine, or stimulate muscle growth. In fact, a high intake of protein from supplements or from foods may contribute to dehydration and could actually hurt athletic performance. The fuel used by muscles for lifting weights is carbohydrate. If too much carbohydrate is replaced by protein, muscle and liver glycogen stores will be low and endurance compromised.

ARE AMINO ACID SUPPLEMENTS ERGOGENIC?

Many amino acid supplements are promoted to athletes by claiming to boost the body's natural production of hormones that stimulate protein synthesis. For example, the amino acids ornithine, arginine, and lysine are marketed with the promise that they will stimulate the release of growth hormone and, in turn, enhance the growth of muscles. Research, however, does not support a beneficial effect on hormonal profile, body composition, muscle size, or exercise performance when oral amino acid supplements are taken at the dose recommended by commercial supplements.[19]

Amino acid supplements are also marketed for a number of other reasons. Glycine supplements are promoted because glycine is a precursor to creatine, but it does not provide the ergogenic effects that creatine supplements do. Glutamine supplements supposedly increase muscle glycogen deposition following intense exercise, enhance immune function, and prevent the adverse effects of over-training such as fatigue and increased incidence of certain infections. Research has not supported these claims. Glutamine has not been found to increase glycogen synthesis.[20] Glutamine is important for immune system cells, and decreases in the plasma glutamine have been reported following prolonged exercise; however, the effects of glutamine supplementation on immune function or the symptoms of overtraining are inconsistent.[18]

The branched-chain amino acids (leucine, isoleucine, and valine) are the predominant amino acids used for fuel during exercise. Supplements of these are promoted to improve performance in endurance athletes. The results of studies examining the effect of branched-chain amino acids on endurance performance have found that they do not enhance performance, particularly when compared to the endurance-enhancing effect of carbohydrate supplementation.[21]

There is little evidence to support the use of amino acid supplements by athletes, and, in general, these supplements are not recommended. High doses of individual amino acids may interfere with the absorption of other amino acids from the diet. There have also been several reports of illness caused by contaminants in the supplements.

DOES CARNITINE HELP YOU BURN FAT?

If you could get fat into your muscle mitochondria faster, you could use it for energy more efficiently. This is what supplements of carnitine claim to do. Carnitine supplements are marketed to athletes as a "fat burner"—a substance that will enhance the utilization of fat during exercise. Fat burners are supposed to increase the use of body fat, spare carbohydrates, and allow athletes to exercise for a longer time before exhaustion. Carnitine is a molecule made from the amino acids lysine and methionine. It is needed to transport fatty acids into the mitochondria, where they are used to produce ATP, but it is not an essential nutrient and does not need to be supplied in the diet to ensure the efficient use of fatty acids. Adequate amounts of carnitine are maintained in the muscle during exercise and supplements have not been found to increase fat loss, the utilization of fat as fuel during exercise, or exercise endurance.[22]

WHAT ABOUT MEDIUM CHAIN TRIGLYCERIDES?

Higher levels of fatty acids in the blood increase the availability of fat as a fuel during exercise. If more fat is available, you use less glucose, sparing glycogen so you can exercise longer. This is the idea behind supplements of **medium chain triglycerides** (**MCTs**). These triglycerides provide medium chain fatty acids, which contain only 8 to 10 carbons in their carbon chain. They are water-soluble, so they can be absorbed directly into the blood, where they are available for use by muscle cells. Typical dietary triglycerides are made up primarily of long chain fatty acids. These must be absorbed into the lymphatic system before even reaching the bloodstream, so they do not cause as great a rise in blood fatty acid levels. Medium chain fatty acids also cross cell membranes easily and can enter the mitochondria for oxidation without the help of carnitine. Triglycerides that provide medium chain fatty acids are marketed to athletes to burn fat, provide an energy source, spare glycogen, and help build muscle. Although the rise in plasma fatty acids that occurs after ingestion of these MCTs might be expected to spare glycogen during high-intensity aerobic exercise, research has not indicated that supplementation with MCTs increases endurance, spares glycogen, or enhances performance.[23, 24]

DOES CREATINE BOOST PERFORMANCE?

Want more quick energy? To get it, many athletes experiment with **creatine** supplements. Creatine is a nitrogen-containing compound found in the body, primarily in muscle, where it is used to make creatine phosphate. It is synthesized by the kidneys, liver, pancreas, and other tissues and is consumed in the diet in meat and milk. The more creatine in the diet, the greater the muscle stores. Supplements of creatine claim to increase the amount of creatine and creatine phosphate in the muscle, increase short-duration, high-power performance, increase muscle mass, and delay fatigue.

Research has demonstrated that supplements of creatine monohydrate increase levels of both creatine and creatine phosphate in muscle.[25] Increasing muscle creatine and creatine phosphate provides muscles with more quick energy for activity, delays fatigue, prevents the accumulation of lactic acid, and allows creatine phosphate to be regenerated more quickly after exercise.[26] These effects make creatine supplementation beneficial for exercise that requires explosive bursts of energy, such as sprinting and weight lifting. Oral creatine supplementation combined with resistance training increases the maximal weight lifted by young men.[27] Creatine supplements have also been found to increase body mass mostly through lean tissue. This increase is believed to be due to water retention related to creatine uptake in the muscle. An increase in muscle mass and strength may also occur in response to the greater amount and intensity of training that may be achieved.[25] Creatine is not beneficial for long-term endurance activities such as marathons.

A number of studies have suggested that creatine supplements are safe, but controlled toxicology studies have not been done and the safety and efficacy of the long-term use of high-dose supplements is unknown.[28] Product purity is also a concern. Because large doses of 5–30 g (1–6 tsp) are needed to be effective, even a minor contaminant might be consumed in significant amounts. Ingestion of creatine before or during exercise is not recommended, and the FDA has advised consumers to consult a physician before using creatine.

IS BICARBONATE A BUFFER BOOSTER?

If you could neutralize the lactic acid produced in your muscles during intense exercise, you could exercise longer. Acid in the muscle affects muscle function and leads to fatigue. Preventing acid accumulation would therefore delay fatigue and improve performance. **Bicarbonate** supplementation has been hypothesized to neutralize the lactic acid that accumulates during anaerobic metabolism. Bicarbonate ions act as buffers in the body. Buffers prevent changes in acidity. Taking sodium bicarbonate, which is just plain baking soda, before exercise has been found to improve performance and delay exhaustion in sports such as sprint cycling, that involve intense exercise lasting only 1 to 7 minutes, but it is of no benefit for lower-intensity aerobic exercise.[18] However, just because baking soda is a common ingredient in the kitchen doesn't make it risk-free. Many people experience abdominal cramps and diarrhea after taking sodium bicarbonate and other possible side effects have not been carefully researched.

CAFFEINE: COFFEE TO GO—LONGER AND FARTHER

Will drinking a cup of coffee help you run farther? Caffeine is a stimulant found in coffee and many soft drinks. It is used as an ergogenic aid because it enhances the release of fatty acids. When fatty acids are used as a fuel source, glycogen is spared, delaying the onset of fatigue. Caffeine has, in fact, been shown to enhance performance during prolonged moderate-intensity endurance exercise and short-term intense exercise.[29] One cup of coffee is not enough, but drinking 2.5 cups of percolated coffee up to an hour before exercising has been shown to improve endurance. The benefits of caffeine, however, differ among individuals. Athletes who are unaccustomed to caffeine consumption respond better than those who consume it on a routine basis. Caffeine is also a diuretic, so, in some athletes, it may impair performance by increasing water loss through urine or by causing gastrointestinal upset. Regardless of its effectiveness, athletes should know that excess caffeine may be illegal. The International Olympic Committee prohibits athletes from competing when urine caffeine levels are 12 µg per ml or

FACT BOX 6.2

How Much Caffeine Is in Your Cup?

Caffeine is the world's most popular drug. The white, bitter-tasting, crystalline substance was first isolated from coffee in 1820. Both words, *caffeine* and *coffee*, are derived from the Arabic word *qahweh* (pronounced "kahveh" in Turkish). It is found naturally in coffee beans, tea leaves, cocoa beans, and cola nuts; it is often added to carbonated beverages and nonprescription medications. Caffeine stimulates the brain and affects behavior. The use of 75–150 mg of caffeine elevates neural activity in many parts of the brain, postpones fatigue, and enhances performance at simple intellectual tasks and at physical work that involves endurance but not fine motor coordination. In the United States, 75% of caffeine is consumed in coffee and 15% in tea. The table below shows how much caffeine you are getting from different types of coffee and other foods and beverages.

Beverage or Food	Caffeine (mg)
Starbucks™ coffee, grande (16 oz)	550
Starbucks™ latte or cappuccino, grande (16 oz)	70
Regular Coffee (7 oz)	80–175
Espresso (1.5 oz)	100
Decaf Coffee, brewed (7 oz)	3–4
Tea, brewed (7 oz)	40–60
Jolt™ Cola (12 oz)	100
Mountain Dew™ (regular or diet, 12 oz)	55
Cola (regular or diet, 12 oz)	40–46
7-Up™ (regular or diet, 12 oz)	0
Hershey™ Bar (1.55 oz)	11
Dark Dove™ Chocolate (1.5 oz)	23
Excedrin™ (2 caplets)	130
Vivarin™ (2 caplets)	400

greater. For urine caffeine to reach this level, an individual would need to drink 6 to 8 cups of coffee within about a 2-hour period. Caffeine is also found in pill form in products such as NoDoz™, which contains about 100 mg of caffeine per tablet—about the same amount as there is in a cup of coffee.

RIBOSE FOR ENERGY?

Ribose is a sugar that is needed to synthesize RNA (ribonucleic acid) and ATP. Ribose supplements claim to increase the synthesis of ATP, improve high-power performance, speed recovery from exercise, and help restore energy levels in the heart and skeletal muscles quickly. Although ribose supplements have been shown to increase ATP production in patients with heart conditions, supplements of ribose have not been found to have any ergogenic effect in healthy people.[30, 31]

CAN HMB PROTECT YOUR MUSCLES?

Exercise is good for your health, but it does cause some muscle damage. Supplements of **Beta-hydroxy-beta-methylbutyrate** or **HMB** claim to prevent or slow muscle damage and blunt muscle breakdown associated with intense physical effort. Beta-hydroxy-beta-methylbutyrate is a compound generated from the breakdown of the amino acid leucine. It is found in some foods and is synthesized in the body. Research in animals and in cells grown in the laboratory has shown that it decreases protein breakdown and increases the breakdown of fat. Short-term studies on the effects of HMB supplements indicate that it decreases muscle breakdown during resistance training and that it improves strength and increases fat-free mass. It is unclear, however, if these effects continue if supplements are used for more than a few months, and it is not clear whether the increase in lean body mass is due to changes in the amount of protein, bone, or water.[32]

WILL GINSENG KEEP YOU GOING?

Ginseng is an herbal supplement promoted to increase endurance. Human clinical trials have shown that when taken in appropriate doses for long enough, Chinese ginseng (*P. ginseng*) may increase muscle strength and aerobic capacity.[33] The benefits may be greater for untrained or older subjects. Although its benefit to endurance is not conclusive, ginseng has certainly passed the test of time. It has been used for over 2,000 years. Ginseng supplements are generally considered safe based on this long history and the few reported side effects. Side effects, however, may occur in some individuals, and ginseng may increase the effects and side effects of other stimulants, such as caffeine. [33]

EPHEDRA: BANNED BY THE FDA

Ephedrine is the active ingredient in **ephedra**, a naturally occurring substance derived from the Chinese herb *Ma huang*. Ephedrine is a stimulant that mimics the effects of epinephrine, causing increases in blood pressure and heart rate. For years, ephedrine-containing supplements were marketed to increase body fat loss, improve athletic performance, and sharpen concentration. Research supports an association between short-term use of ephedrine and increased weight loss (compared to placebo).[34] The data support a modest effect of ephedrine plus caffeine on very short-term athletic performance but no studies have assessed the sustained use of ephedrine on performance over time.[34] Despite these potential benefits, ephedrine use has been associated with serious side effects, including nervousness, headaches, nausea, hypertension, cardiac arrhythmias, heart attack, stroke, and even death. Products containing ephedra accounted for 64% of all adverse reactions to herbs in the United States, yet these products represent less than 1% of herbal product sales.[35] Because of health risks associated with the use of ephedra, the sale of ephedra-containing supplements was banned by the FDA as of April 12, 2004.

ANABOLIC STEROIDS BULK YOU UP *ILLEGALLY*

Is it worth risking your health to have bigger muscles? Unfortunately, some athletes may still be willing to sacrifice their health for the benefits that **anabolic steroids** provide. The term *anabolic steroid* refers to steroid hormones that accelerate protein synthesis and growth. The anabolic steroids used by athletes are synthetic versions of the human steroid hormone testosterone. Natural testosterone stimulates and maintains the male sexual organs and promotes the development of bones and muscles and the growth of skin and hair.

FACT BOX 6.3

The Dangers of Ephedra

Ephedra is an herbal extract that was used for years in dietary supplements that promised to reduce appetite or improve athletic performance. There is some evidence that it had some benefits, particulary for weight loss, but it can also have serious side effects, including heart attack, stroke, and even death. Eventually, the FDA concluded that the dangers of ephedra outweighed its benefits; ephedra became the first dietary supplement to be banned by the FDA.

The risks of ephedra were dramatically demonstrated in February 2003 when 23-year-old baseball pitcher Steve Belcher died of heat stroke while taking an ephedra-containing supplement to lose weight. He collapsed during a training session in the hot, humid Florida weather and died the next day when his body temperature reached 108°F. An autopsy revealed ephedra in his blood, along with smaller amounts of two other stimulants—pseudoephedrine and caffeine. Did ephedra cause Steve's death? No one can be sure that he wouldn't have died even if he hadn't taken it. Steve was overweight and out of shape. He was not acclimated to the weather. He was on a weight-loss diet and did not feel well or eat the night before he collapsed. He also had high blood pressure and abnormal liver function tests. These were certainly all factors in his death, but ephedra constricts blood vessels in the skin and raises body temperature, perhaps by up to 2°F. So, even though the cause of death was heat stroke, ephedra may well have played a role. This would not be the first case of a serious problem associated with this supplement. A review of 16,000 reports of adverse effects revealed two deaths, four heart attacks, nine strokes, one seizure, and five psychiatric cases involving ephedra. Even before the FDA ordered ephedra-containing supplements off the shelves, ephedra had been banned by minor league baseball, the NFL, NCAA, and the International Olympic Committee.

The synthetic testosterone used by athletes has a greater effect on muscle development and on bone, skin, and hair than it does on sexual organs. When synthetic testosterone is taken in conjunction with exercise and an adequate diet, muscle mass does increase. However, because these drugs increase body levels of testosterone, production of natural testosterone is reduced. Without natural testosterone, the sexual organs are not maintained; this leads to testicular shrinkage and a decrease in sperm production. In adolescents, the use of synthetic testosterone causes bone growth to stop and height to be stunted. Anabolic steroid use may also cause oily skin and acne, water retention in the tissues, yellowing of the eyes and skin, coronary artery disease, liver disease, and sometimes death. In addition to these physiological effects, users may have psychological and behavioral side effects such as violent outbursts and depression, possibly leading to suicide. The dangers of steroid use are increased by the fact that they are illegal, so their manufacturing and distribution procedures are not regulated. Users can never be sure of the potency and purity of what they are taking.

ARE STEROID PRECURSORS ANY SAFER THAN ANABOLIC STEROIDS?

Steroid precursors may sound like the perfect alternative to anabolic steroids. These are compounds that can be converted into steroid hormones in the body. They include androstenedione, androstenediol, DHEA, norandrostenediol, and norandrostenedione. They are often marketed as an alternative to anabolic steroids to increase muscle mass. Many steroid precursors can be sold legally as dietary supplements. But do they work, and are they safe?

The best known of the steroid precursors is androstenedione, often referred to as "andro." It is a precursor to testosterone and is marketed to increase levels of testosterone. Andro has been used for years by bodybuilders, but it was launched to public prominence when major league baseball player Mark McGwire announced his use of it during the 1998 major league baseball season when he hit 70 home runs, breaking the league's single-season home-run record. McGwire has subsequently stopped using andro.

Did andro help McGuire hit all those home runs? No one can know for sure, but there is evidence that andro has anabolic effects if taken in sufficient amounts for a long enough time. It is converted into estrogen and testosterone in the body and, if enough is taken, blood levels of these hormones increase.[36] If levels increase enough to have anabolic effects, then so do the risks associated with high levels of anabolic steroids. The risks are greatest in children and adolescents. They include disruption of sexual developement, testicular shrinkage, stunted growth, and liver and heart disease. In March 2004, in response to concerns about the safety of this steroid precursor, the FDA told companies to stop selling the supplements containing andro unless they can prove that it is not dangerous.

DHEA is another steroid precursor. DHEA supplements claim to increase testosterone production, boost the immune system, preserve youth, and decrease joint pain and fatigue, but there is no data to support any ergogenic effects.

PEPTIDE HORMONES ARE BY PRESCRIPTION ONLY

Peptide hormones are hormones made from chains of amino acids. The ability to produce peptide hormones through genetic engineering has increased their availability not only to individuals with conditions that require these hormones, but also to athletes. These hormones are illegal if not prescribed by a physician and most have dangerous side effects. It is difficult to detect these drugs in athletes because they are present naturally and are broken down rapidly and little is excreted in the urine.

Does Growth Hormone Grow Muscles?

Human **growth hormone** is a peptide hormone that is produced by the pituitary gland. It is important for tissue building during childhood growth. Genetically engineered growth hormone is used to treat children who are small due to growth hormone deficiency. In adults, growth hormone maintains lean tissue, stimulates fat breakdown, increases the number of red blood cells, and boosts heart function. This hormone is appealing to athletes because it increases muscle protein synthesis. Despite these physiological effects, the ergogenic benefits of growth hormone among athletes remain unproven. More important, prolonged use of growth hormone can cause heart dysfunction and high blood pressure as well as excessive growth of some body parts, such as hands, feet, and facial features.

Erythropoietin (EPO): The Blood Booster

Another peptide hormone that is popular among endurance athletes is **erythropoietin**, known as EPO. Natural erythropoietin is produced by the kidneys and stimulates stem cells in the bone marrow to differentiate into red blood cells. Genetically engineered EPO is used to treat anemia due to kidney disease, chemotherapy, HIV infection, and blood loss. It can enhance the performance of endurance athletes by increasing the number of red blood cells and, hence, the ability to transport oxygen to the muscles. It therefore increases VO_2max and aerobic performance and spares glycogen. However, too much EPO can cause the production of too many red blood cells, which can lead to excessive blood clotting, heart attacks, and strokes. The International Olympic Committee banned EPO in 1990 after it was linked to the death of more than a dozen cyclists.[37]

OTHER SUPPLEMENTS

The list of things athletes will ingest to enhance performance is endless. It includes such substances as bee pollen, brewer's yeast, wheat germ oil, royal jelly, and DNA and RNA.

Bee pollen is a mixture of the pollen of flowering plants, plant nectar, and bee saliva. It contains no extraordinary factors and has not been shown to have any performance-enhancing effects. In addition, ingesting or inhaling bee pollen can be hazardous to individuals who are allergic to various plant pollens.[38]

Brewer's yeast is a source of B vitamins and some minerals, but has not been demonstrated to have any ergogenic properties. Likewise, there is no evidence to support claims that wheat germ oil will aid endurance. As an oil, it is high in fat, but it is no better as an energy source than any other fat.

Royal jelly is a substance produced by worker bees to feed the queen bee. Although it helps the queen bee grow to twice the size of worker bees and to live 40 times longer, royal jelly does not appear to enhance athletic capacity in humans.

Finally, DNA and RNA are marketed to aid in tissue regeneration. In the body, they carry genetic information and are needed to synthesize proteins, but DNA and RNA are not required in the diet, and supplements do not help replace damaged cells.

CONNECTIONS

Anything designed to enhance performance can be considered an ergogenic aid. If anything, these products often provide more of a psychological advantage than a physiological edge. Dietary supplements marketed as ergogenic aids include vitamins, minerals, proteins, amino acids, lipids, herbs, hormones, and substances made by the body. Some, such as antioxidant supplements, are relatively harmless but have not been shown to enhance performance. Others, such as creatine, bicarbonate, and caffeine are not associated with serious side effects and may enhance performance in certain types of activities. Some others, such as anabolic steroids and EPO, can enhance performance but are extremely dangerous to your health. Certain substances, in fact, can prevent an athlete from reaching his or her maximal level of performance. Many ergogenic supplements are illegal in both amateur and professional athletics. When considering the use of an ergogenic supplement, it is important to weigh the health risks against potential benefits. Just because a product is sold doesn't make it safe, and just because something appears in print does not make it true. Choosing to use an ergogenic aid should be a serious decision that is discussed with your doctor. Many of these supplements have dangerous interactions with other medications and can exacerbate existent health conditions.

7

Nutritional Problems Common Among Athletes

Sometimes, in an effort to improve performance or achieve unrealistic goals, athletes may consume unhealthy diets or push their bodies too hard. The consequences may actually end up hurting performance.

LOSING AND GAINING WEIGHT

How much you weigh can affect your speed, endurance, and power; how much muscle and fat you have can influence your strength, agility, and appearance. Athletes often try to lose or gain weight to optimize their performance. Those involved in activities like gymnastics and certain running events, in which small, lean bodies offer an advantage, may restrict energy intake to maintain a low body weight. Athletes involved in sports such as football or rugby may try to increase body weight and strength to give them a

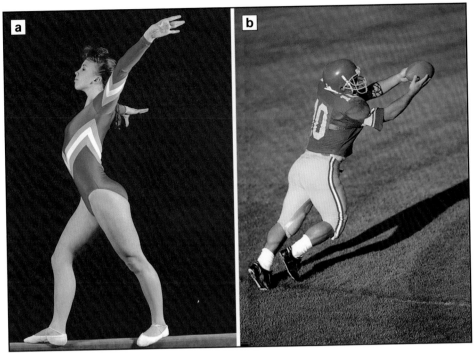

Figure 7.1 Different body composition is appropriate for different sports. Although both gymnasts and football players have significant muscle mass, gymnasts (a) are usually thin and lean, while football players (b) are generally more bulky. These very different body types are advantageous in different sports.

competitive advantage. Those involved in sports with weight classes may aim for a specific weight to be at the top of a lower weight class (Figure 7.1).

Concern about body weight and composition may lead to unhealthy weight-loss practices or may precipitate eating disorders. Regardless of their sport, athletes should aim for a healthy weight. This is a weight that can realistically be maintained, allows for improvement in exercise performance, minimizes the chance of injury or illness, and reduces the risk of chronic disease. Weight changes, whether to increase or decrease body weight, should be accomplished slowly in the off-season or at the beginning of the season, before competition begins.

How to Gain Weight Safely

To gain weight, you need to increase your intake by 500 to 1,000 calories per day. Strength training should be increased to ensure that you primarily gain lean tissue. The rate of weight gain will depend on your genetic makeup, how many extra calories you consume, and the type of training program you follow.

How to Lose Weight Safely

To lose weight and remain healthy, you need to reduce energy intake enough to allow gradual weight loss while maintaining a healthy diet. A decrease of 10–20% of normal calorie intake will allow weight loss without making you feel deprived or hungry. For example, if an athlete's normal intake is 3,000 calories per day, decreasing this by 300 to 600 calories should cause a slow weight loss. To preserve lean body mass and enhance fat loss, weight loss should take place at a rate of about 1/2 to 2 pounds per week and activity levels should be maintained. Dieting to maintain an unrealistically low weight may threaten nutritional status, health, and athletic performance.

The Dangers of "Making Weight"

"Making weight" refers to the practice of keeping weight at a specific level to fit into a set weight category. For example, sports with weight classes such as wrestling may require an athlete to gain or lose weight to fit into a particular category. Competing at the high end of a weight class is believed to give the athlete an advantage over smaller opponents. But weight changes are not necessarily beneficial to the individual athlete's health or performance. Often, athletes use dehydration to reduce weight rapidly. This is accomplished through practices such as vigorous exercise, fluid restriction, exercising while wearing vapor-impermeable suits, and sitting in hot environments such as saunas and steam rooms. More extreme measures include intentional vomiting and the use of diuretics and laxatives. These practices can be dangerous and even fatal. They may impair performance and can adversely affect heart and kidney function, temperature regulation, and electrolyte balance.[39] Athletes often think they can dehydrate for the weigh-in and then rehydrate in time for competition, but the time between weigh-in and competition is not sufficient for fluid and electrolyte balance to return to normal in the muscles, or for the replenishment of muscle and liver glycogen.[40]

EATING DISORDERS: ATHLETES AT RISK

Eating disorders are a group of conditions that are characterized by a pathological concern with body weight and shape. They are primarily psychological disorders but they also involve nutrition-related behaviors and complications. Athletes are under extreme pressure to achieve and maintain a body weight that optimizes their performance. Failure to meet weight-loss goals may have serious consequences, such as being cut from the team or restricted from competition. This pressure may cause athletes to follow strict diets and maintain body weights that are not healthy. This, combined with the self-motivation and discipline that characterizes successful athletes, makes many vulnerable to eating disorders.

FACT BOX 7.1

Why Did Three Young Wrestlers Die?

In 1997, during a period of a little over a month, three young wrestlers died while trying to "make weight."[a] They were exercising while wearing rubber suits to sweat off enough water to qualify for a lighter weight class. The deaths were caused by an increase in blood potassium concentration, which stops the heart. Muscle fibers that are damaged by heat release potassium. Normally, potassium levels in the blood are precisely regulated, but with dehydration, blood flow through the kidneys is reduced. It is possible that some type of medication or supplement also played a role, but exercising in the heat is dangerous and, as a result of these deaths, wrestling weight classes were altered to eliminate the lightest weight class, plastic sweatsuits were banned, wrestling room temperatures could be no warmer than 75°F, weigh-ins have been moved to one hour before competition, and mandatory weight-loss rules have been put in place, restricting the amount of weight that can be lost.

a. Available online at *http://www.cin.org/archives/cinhealth/199901/0044.htm.*

Athletes With Anorexia

One type of eating disorder that may occur among athletes is **anorexia nervosa**. Anorexia nervosa is diagnosed by the loss of 15% or more of the body weight. This is accomplished by restricting food intake and using behaviors such as vomiting after eating, abuse of laxatives, and excessive exercise to eliminate or use up calories. Individuals with anorexia are generally very secretive about their eating behaviors. An athlete's regimented schedule makes it easy for him or her to use training diets and timetables, travel, or competition as an excuse not to eat normally. Over time, the continued starvation characteristic of anorexia leads to serious health problems as well as a decline in athletic performance. Starvation can lead to abnormal heart rhythms, low blood pressure, and atrophy of the heart muscle. The lack of food means that there is not adequate energy and nutrients to support activity and growth. Sleep disorders are also common in people with anorexia.

Binging and Purging: Bulimia

The eating disorder **bulimia nervosa** is more common than anorexia. It is characterized by a cycle of binging and purging. *Binging* is the rapid consumption of a large amount of food, which is accompanied by feelings of guilt and shame. *Purging* refers to methods used to eliminate excess calories from the body. These include self-induced vomiting, misuse of laxatives and diuretics, as well as excessive dieting and exercise. Bulimia may begin because an athlete is unable to stick to a restrictive diet or because the hunger associated with a very low-calorie diet leads to binging. Those with bulimia are usually of normal or slightly higher than normal body weight. Most of the health complications associated with bulimia, including tooth decay from repeating vomiting and dangerous changes in body chemistry, are a result of the binge-purge cycle.

Compulsive Exercising

The use of compulsive exercise to control weight has less to do with food than either anorexia or bulimia, but it is nonetheless considered an eating disorder as well. Compulsive exercisers use extreme training as a way to purge calories. This behavior is easy to justify because it is a common belief that serious athletes can never work too hard or too long, and pain is accepted as an indicator of achievement. Compulsive exercisers will force themselves to exercise even when they don't feel well and may miss social events in order to fulfill their exercise quota. They often calculate exercise goals based on how much they eat. They believe that any break in the training schedule will cause them to gain weight and make their performance suffer. Compulsive exercise can lead to more serious eating disorders such as anorexia and bulimia and may also bring on severe health problems, including kidney failure, heart attack, and death.

THE FEMALE ATHLETE TRIAD

In female athletes, the desire to reduce body weight and fat to improve performance, achieve an ideal body image, and meet goals set by coaches, trainers, or parents increases the risk for a syndrome of interrelated disorders referred to as the **female athlete triad**. This syndrome includes disordered eating, **amenorrhea**, and **osteoporosis**. These often occur together because the combination of low energy intake from eating disorders and high level of energy output from exercise causes alterations in the secretion of reproductive hormones. This may lead to the delayed onset or absence of menstruation, referred to as amenorrhea. Amenorrhea is accompanied by low levels of the hormone estrogen, which is needed for bone

---

FACT BOX 7.2

The Risk of Eating Disorders Is Greater in Some Sports

Ninety-three percent of eating disorders among athletes involve women's sports. The most problematic are women's cross country, women's gymnastics, women's swimming, and women's track and field events. The male sports with the highest number of participants with eating disorders are wrestling and cross country.[a]

a. From ANRED (Anorexia Nervosa and Related Eating Disorders, Inc.). "Athletes with eating disorders: An overview." Available online at http://www.anred.com/ath_intro.html.

health. Low estrogen decreases calcium absorption from the diet and causes reductions in bone mass and bone-mineral density. Female athletes also tend to have low calcium intakes. The combination of low estrogen levels and poor calcium intake leads to premature bone loss, failure to reach a healthy bone mass, and an increased risk of bone fractures (osteoporosis). Exercise, particularly weight-bearing exercise, generally increases bone density, thereby reducing the risk of osteoporosis. However, when estrogen levels are low due to amenorrhea, neither adequate dietary calcium nor the increase in bone mass brought about by weight-bearing exercise can compensate for bone loss. If menses resume, bone loss can at least be partially reversed, but whether these athletes are at greater risk for osteoporosis later in life is not known[41] (Figure 7.2).

MORE ISN'T ALWAYS BETTER: OVERTRAINING SYNDROME

Most athletes believe that training harder improves their performance, but this isn't always the case. It turns out that enough rest is just as important as enough training. Muscle strength and cardiovascular and respiratory fitness improve in response to the stress of exercise training. Initially, training can cause fatigue and weakness, but during rest periods, the body rebuilds to become stronger. If not enough rest occurs between exercise sessions, there is no time to regenerate, so fitness and performance do not improve. In competitive athletes, excessive training can lead to **overtraining syndrome**, which involves emotional, behavioral, and physical symptoms that persist for weeks to months. It is caused by repeatedly training without sufficient rest to allow for recovery. The most common symptom of overtraining syndrome is fatigue that limits workouts and is felt even at rest. Some athletes experience a decrease in appetite and weight loss as well as muscle soreness, increased frequency of viral illnesses, and higher incidence of injuries. They may become moody, easily irritated, depressed, have altered sleep patterns, or lose their competitive desire and enthusiasm. Although overtraining syndrome occurs only in serious athletes who are working out extensively, rest is essential for anyone who is trying to improve fitness.

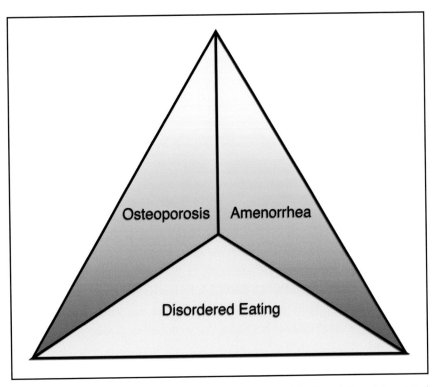

Figure 7.2 The female athlete triad is a dangerous combination of three interrelated disorders: eating disorders, the stop of menstruation (amenorrhea), and osteoporosis (the degeneration of bones). The root cause of the triad—disordered eating—causes problems that affect all aspects of a woman's physical health.

LOW IRON MEANS POOR PERFORMANCE

Low iron stores, referred to as iron depletion, are one of the most prevalent nutritional problems seen in athletes, particularly female athletes. If this condition progresses to iron deficiency anemia, it can impair exercise performance as well as reduce immune function and affect other physiological processes.[42]

Low iron stores may be caused by an inadequate dietary iron intake, a rise in the body's demand for iron, increased iron losses, or a redistribution of iron due to exercise training. Dietary iron intake may be low in athletes who are attempting to keep body weight low, or in those who consume a vegetarian diet and therefore do not eat meat. Meat is an excellent source of readily absorbable iron. Iron needs may be increased in athletes because exercise stimulates the production of red blood cells, so more iron is needed for hemoglobin synthesis. Iron is also needed for the synthesis of muscle myoglobin and the iron-containing proteins needed for ATP production in the mitochondria. Prolonged training may also increase iron losses, possibly because of increased fecal, urinary, and sweat losses. Iron balance may also be affected by the breaking of red blood cells from impact in events such as running (foot-strike hemolysis) or by the contraction of large muscles. However, this rarely causes anemia because the breaking of red blood cells stimulates the production of new ones.[43]

Some athletes experience a condition known as sports anemia, which is a temporary decrease in hemoglobin concentration that occurs during exercise training. It occurs when the blood volume expands to increase oxygen delivery, but the synthesis of red blood cells lags behind the increase in plasma volume. This is an adaptation to training and does not seem to impair delivery of oxygen to tissues.

VEGETARIAN DIETS FOR ATHLETES

Vegetarian diets exclude or partially exclude animal products. These diets are generally healthy but may increase the risk of certain

---

FACT BOX 7.3

Swimming Half the Time

We usually think that more training means greater increases in strength and endurance and an overall improvement in performance. The fact that this is not always the case was demonstrated by a study involving swimmers. Half the swimmers trained for an hour and a half in the morning and again for an hour and a half in the afternoon. The other group of swimmers only participated in the afternoon training session. The swimmers who trained twice as much experienced a decline in speed, while the other group showed improvement. Doubling the training did not enhance the performance.[a]

a. Costill, D.L., R. Thomas, R.A. Robergs, et al. "Adaptations to swimming training: Influence of training volume." *Medicine and Science in Sports and Exercise* 23 (1991): 371–377.

nutritional problems when consumed by athletes. Athletes often have very high energy requirements. Although in most cases it is easy to meet energy needs by eating a vegetarian diet, energy availability may be reduced if the diet is very high in fiber. The best way to determine if energy needs are being met by the diet is to monitor body weight and composition.

Vegetarian diets tend to be lower in protein than are diets that contain animal products. Although the quality of the protein in vegetarian diets is adequate for adults, the plant proteins are not as easily digested. To compensate for this, an increase in protein intake of about 10% can be made. Therefore, vegetarian athletes should consume 1.3–1.8 grams of protein per kilogram of body weight— the equivalent of 90–130 grams of protein for a 150-pound (68-kg) person.[7] Athletes with relatively low energy requirements need to choose foods carefully to ensure that their protein intakes meet these recommendations.

Vegetarian athletes may be at risk for low intake of a number of vitamins and minerals, including vitamin B_{12}, vitamin D, riboflavin, iron, calcium, and zinc. The best dietary sources of these nutrients are animal products. As discussed above, iron is of particular concern to the athlete. The iron in plant foods is not absorbed as efficiently as that found in animal foods. Vegetarians tend to have lower iron stores than nonvegetarians, even when iron intake is the same. Given that exercise may increase iron needs, vegetarian athletes, especially women, are at greater risk of low iron status.

Some athletes, especially women, may switch to a vegetarian diet as a means to lose weight and attain a leaner body. This can, in some cases, indicate that the athlete is at risk for developing an eating disorder.

CONNECTIONS

In an effort to improve performance, athletes may engage in certain practices, such as restricting food intake or training excessively, that increase the possibility of injury or illness. Health problems often occur as a result of attempts to lose or gain body weight. Severe weight-loss diets and the use of dehydration to achieve short-term weight loss can impair health and performance. Some athletes who are concerned about their weight may develop eating disorders. When these occur in women in combination with amenorrhea and osteoporosis, it is referred to as female athlete triad. This syndrome has long-term consequences for bone health. Excessive training can lead to overtraining syndrome, which is characterized by fatigue that limits workouts, makes viral illnesses more frequent, and increases the incidence of injuries. Iron deficiency is also a common problem in athletes, particularly females. Poor iron status may be caused by an inadequate iron intake, an increased demand for iron, increased iron losses, or a redistribution of iron due to exercise training. Some athletes may be at risk for deficiencies of iron, calcium, vitamin B_{12}, vitamin D, riboflavin, and zinc because they eat vegetarian diets. In order to maintain health while remaining physically active, it is important to follow a diet that meets nutrient needs and to keep training at a reasonable level.

8

Diet and Exercise for a Healthy Life

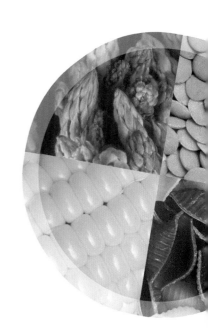

A healthy lifestyle can keep you feeling fit and energetic and looking lean. It can also reduce the chances that you will develop a chronic degenerative disease as you age. A proper diet and regular exercise are part of this healthy lifestyle; learning to choose foods wisely and incorporating exercise into your daily routine can help you live a long and healthy life.

THE BENEFITS OF A HEALTHY LIFESTYLE

Four of the leading causes of death in the United States today are heart disease, stroke, cancer, and diabetes; all of these diseases are related to diet and lifestyle. Together, they account for about two-thirds of all deaths in the United States each year. Your genetic makeup is an important determinant of your risk for developing these diseases, but lifestyle choices such as a poor diet, lack of exercise, smoking, and alcohol abuse also play a vital role. You cannot control what genes you inherit, but you can control what foods you eat and how much exercise you get.

The right choices can reduce your risk of developing degenerative diseases and may slow the progression of any conditions you already have.

A healthy diet and a regular exercise program make it easier to maintain an appropriate body weight and help keep muscles, bones, and joints healthy. They can help prevent or delay the onset of heart disease, high blood pressure, diabetes, cancer, and osteoporosis. In addition to protecting you from chronic diseases, a nutritious diet helps promote a strong immune system, which protects you from infectious diseases as well as cancer. Exercise also has psychological benefits that can help prevent depression and improve mood, sleep patterns, and overall outlook on life.

A Healthy Body Weight

A suitable body weight is associated with health and longevity. Carrying excess body fat increases the risk of heart disease, diabetes, stroke, gallbladder disease, sleep disorders, respiratory problems, and some types of cancer. Maintaining weight at a proper level reduces the risk of these diseases. For athletes, a healthy weight can also optimize performance.

Diet and exercise are both essential for maintaining weight because calorie intake must be balanced with calorie use. Choosing a diet that is rich in whole grains, fruits, and vegetables and moderate in fat can make balancing intake with expenditure easier. Regular exercise helps because it increases energy expenditure and thereby allows you to consume more food without gaining weight. For example, an active 20-year-old woman needs to take in about 500 calories more per day to maintain weight than a sedentary woman of the same age, height, and weight.

Heart Disease

Generally, when we use the term *heart disease*, we are talking about atherosclerosis. This is a condition in which deposits on the walls of the arteries cause them to narrow and lose elasticity.

The risk of developing atherosclerosis is increased by other conditions, including obesity, high blood pressure, high cholesterol levels, and diabetes. It is also increased by lifestyle factors such as cigarette smoking, lack of exercise, and a diet high in saturated fat, cholesterol, and *trans* fat. Diets high in fiber, antioxidants such as vitamins C and E, and fish and plant oils, which are high in monounsaturated and polyunsaturated fats, can reduce the risk of atherosclerosis. A healthy diet plentiful in whole grains, fruits, and vegetables will be naturally low in saturated fat and cholesterol and high in unsaturated fats, fiber, and antioxidants. Adding exercise to this healthy mix further reduces risk. Aerobic exercise decreases the risk of atherosclerosis by strengthening the heart muscle, thereby lowering resting heart rate and decreasing the heart's workload. It can lower blood pressure and increase levels of HDL (healthy) cholesterol in the blood, both of which reduce the risk of atherosclerosis.[44]

High Blood Pressure and Stroke

High blood pressure, or hypertension, can damage the blood vessels. This can increase the risk of atherosclerosis by causing plaque to form on blood vessel walls. If left untreated, high blood pressure may eventually lead to a stroke, which occurs when there is a rupture or blockage of a blood vessel in the brain, shutting off blood flow to part of the brain. Blood pressure is increased by the presence of other diseases, including atherosclerosis, obesity, and diabetes. A healthy diet and exercise can lower blood pressure.

Many nutrients appear to have a role in regulating blood pressure. Salt is perhaps the best known. Diets high in salt are associated with a greater incidence of hypertension, and reducing salt intake can help reduce blood pressure in many people. Low intakes of other nutrients, including calcium, magnesium, and potassium, have been associated with increases in blood pressure. A dietary pattern that is rich in calcium, magnesium, and potassium and moderate in sodium has been shown to help keep blood pressure in the healthy range. Such a pattern is high in fruits and vegetables and provides whole grains, low-fat dairy products, and lean meats. Maintaining a healthy weight is also important for healthy blood pressure; a weight loss of just 10 pounds can significantly lower blood pressure. Exercise helps with weight loss and increasing exercise even without weight loss can directly lower blood pressure by improving cardiovascular fitness and reducing stress.

Diabetes

Being overweight dramatically increases your risk of developing diabetes. Diabetes is a disease in which blood glucose levels are elevated. Many scientists now believe that a dietary pattern that is high in refined carbohydrates such as sugar and refined starches like white bread, pasta, and white rice may also increase the long-term risk of developing diabetes. A diet that is low in refined starches and added sugars from foods like cookies, cakes, and soft drinks may reduce the risk of diabetes. This type of diet also helps maintain body weight in a healthy range. Aerobic exercise can decrease the risk of developing diabetes by keeping body weight healthy and by reducing insulin needs. In people who already have diabetes, exercise can reduce or eliminate the need for medication.

Cancer

A healthy diet and exercise have both been shown to reduce cancer risk. A proper diet is high in vitamins, minerals, and phytochemicals, many of which may protect against cancer development. Part of this protection is due to the antioxidant functions of many phytochemicals and nutrients such as vitamin E, vitamin C, and selenium. Part is due to other protective effects. For instance, vitamin A helps maintain a healthy immune system to help destroy cancer cells. A diet rich in calcium and vitamin D may protect against colon cancer. A diet high in fiber reduces the risk of colon, rectal, and breast cancer. Plenty of fluids may reduce the risk of bladder cancer. Different phytochemicals protect against cancer through mechanisms such as slowing the growth of cancer cells, increasing the activity of enzymes that deactivate cancer-causing substances, helping cells repair themselves, and inhibiting enzymes that activate carcinogens. A healthy diet also promotes the maintenance of a healthy weight, which reduces cancer risk. Individuals who exercise regularly may further reduce their cancer risk. Research has shown that active individuals are less likely to develop colon cancer than are their sedentary counterparts. There is also some evidence that exercise reduces breast cancer risk.

Osteoporosis

Did your parents tell you to drink your milk? That was good advice. Milk is an excellent source of calcium. Adequate calcium throughout life helps you develop dense, strong bones and keep them. This reduces the likelihood that you will develop osteoporosis, a bone disorder that makes bones less dense and more fragile and therefore more likely to break. A healthy diet includes plenty of calcium from low-fat dairy products, leafy green vegetables like spinach, legumes, and fish (such as sardines) eaten with bones. Exercise can prevent osteoporosis because the "use it or lose it" principle applies to bones as well as muscles. Regular weight-bearing exercise such as walking, running, and aerobic dance can increase the density of bones, reducing the risk of osteoporosis. Exercise can also benefit individuals with arthritis because the strength and flexibility promoted by exercise help arthritic joints move more easily.

WHAT IS A HEALTHY DIET?

A healthy diet provides the right number of calories to keep your weight within the desirable range; the proper balance of carbohydrates, protein, and fat choices; plenty of water; and sufficient but not excessive amounts of essential vitamins and minerals. How this translates into specific food choices depends on individual needs and preferences. Whether you are a couch potato or an Olympic hopeful, the recommendations from the Food Guide Pyramid and the Dietary Guidelines can help you choose a proper diet. These guidelines are designed to help you choose a diet that is rich in whole grains, fruits, and vegetables; high in fiber; moderate in fat and sodium; and low in saturated fat, cholesterol, *trans* fat, and added sugars. Eating this diet doesn't mean giving up your favorite foods. But it does require some planning and means that you should choose foods with variety and balance in mind.

Variety is important to a healthy diet because, even within food groups, different foods provide different nutrients. For example, strawberries are a fruit that provides vitamin C but little vitamin A, whereas apricots are a good a source of vitamin A, but provide less vitamin C. If you choose only strawberries, you will get plenty of vitamin C but may be lacking in vitamin A. Balancing your diet means selecting foods that complement each other. This requires considering the nutrient density of foods you choose. Foods low in nutrient density such as baked goods, snack foods, and sodas should be balanced with nutrient-dense choices such as salads, fresh fruit, and large vegetable servings. For one meal, you may choose a burger, french fries, and a milkshake; you can balance this with a salad, brown rice, and chicken at the next meal. By following these recommendations, most people can meet their nutrient needs. For those who have increased needs or limited food choices, fortified foods such as calcium-fortified orange juice and iron-fortified breakfast cereals are available. In some cases, vitamin and mineral supplements can be helpful, but these should be used with caution to avoid taking a toxic amount.

No single dietary component can make or break a diet. Rather, it is the overall pattern of intake combined with lifestyle factors that determines the relationship between your diet and your health. This fact is demonstrated by the dietary pattern in Italy and other Mediterranean countries, where the people consume more fat than U.S. citizens do, yet have a lower incidence of heart disease than that of Americans. This is thought to be related to the fact that much of the fat in this Mediterranean diet is monounsaturated fat from olive oil, that the Mediterranean diet includes more fruits and vegetables, and that the lifestyle there is more active and less stressful than it is in the United States.

HOW MUCH EXERCISE SHOULD YOU GET?

Exercise is good for you, yet most Americans include very little activity in their daily lives. In fact, about 25% of adult Americans claim that they get no physical activity at all during their leisure time[45] (Figure 8.1). A regular program of exercise increases your fitness level and makes the tasks of everyday life easier. As discussed above, regular physical activity can help you keep your

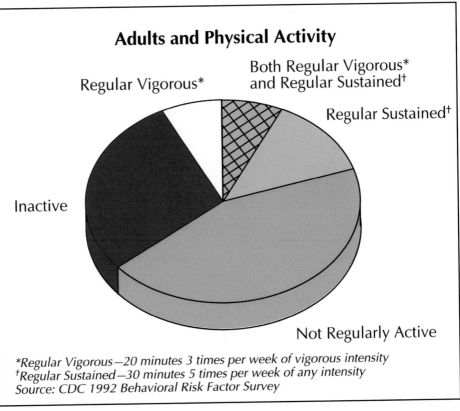

Adults and Physical Activity

Regular Vigorous*

Both Regular Vigorous*
and Regular Sustained†

Regular Sustained†

Inactive

Not Regularly Active

*Regular Vigorous—20 minutes 3 times per week of vigorous intensity
†Regular Sustained—30 minutes 5 times per week of any intensity
Source: CDC 1992 Behavioral Risk Factor Survey

Figure 8.1 Most Americans do not get the recommended amount of exercise. According to this CDC graph, only about 25% of Americans get any regular exercise at all, which is necessary to keep the body healthy. The vast majority of U.S. citizens fall into the "not active" categories.

weight within the healthy range and can help reduce the risk of a variety of chronic diseases. It enhances fitness, strength, flexibility, and body composition, and contributes greatly to an improved quality of life. Exercise also promotes psychological well-being and reduces feelings of depression and anxiety. It stimulates the release of chemicals called endorphins, which are thought to be natural tranquilizers that play a role in triggering what athletes describe as an "exercise high." In addition to causing this state of exercise euphoria, endorphins are believed to reduce anxiety, aid in relaxation, and improve mood, pain tolerance, and appetite control.

In order to get theses benefits, exercise needs to be part of your daily routine. The most recent public health messages recommend 60 minutes of moderate physical activity daily.[46] This is equivalent to walking at a speed of about 3 to 4 miles per hour for 1 hour. The same amount of exercise can be obtained in shorter sessions of more intense activity, such as jogging or playing basketball for 30 minutes (Table 8.1). Less exercise than this is not enough to promote the maintenance of a healthy body weight or to fully reduce chronic disease risk. Higher activity levels do not necessarily enhance other health benefits, and excessive amounts of physical activity can lead to injuries, menstrual abnormalities, and bone weakening.

What Type of Exercise Is Best?

There is no one best type of exercise. As with diet, variety is key. Choose activities you enjoy and mix them up. Bike one day, swim the next, and then spend a session lifting weights at the gym. A well-planned exercise regimen includes aerobic exercise to improve

---

FACT BOX 8.1

How Much Exercise Do You Get?

Americans need to move more. Over 60% of U.S. adults do not engage in the recommended amount of activity, and approximately 25% are not active at all.[a] Women are less active than men, older people are less active than younger ones, African Americans and Hispanics are less active than whites, and less wealthy people are not as active as the affluent. Adults aren't the only ones who need to get off the couch. Nearly half of American youths between age 12 and 21 are not vigorously active on a regular basis and about 14% of young people report no recent physical activity. Participation in all types of physical activity declines strikingly as age or grade in school increases.

a. CDC. "Physical Activity and Health, A Report of the Surgeon General, Fact Sheets." Available online at http://www.cdc.gov/nccdphp/sgr/fact.htm.

Table 8.1—How Much of What Type of Activity

Do these for 60 minutes	Walk briskly
	Play golf, pulling or carrying clubs
	Swim at a recreational pace
	Mow the lawn with a power motor
	Play doubles tennis
	Bicycle at 5 to 9 mph on level terrain or with a few hills
	Scrub floors or wash windows
	Lift weights using hydraulic machines or free weights
Do these for 30 minutes	Racewalk, jog, or run
	Swim laps
	Mow the lawn with a push mower
	Play singles tennis
	Bicycle at more than 10 mph, or on steep uphill terrain
	Move furniture
	Lift weights in circuit training

cardiovascular and respiratory fitness, stretching to promote and maintain flexibility, and resistance training to enhance the strength and endurance of specific muscles.

To decrease the risk of injury, each exercise session should begin with a warm-up to increase blood flow to the muscles. Warm muscles are limber, and keeping muscles loose reduces the risk of injury and soreness. A five-minute warm-up of walking or rhythmic movement is recommended before starting any strenuous activity. A cooldown after the workout helps prevent muscle cramps and slowly brings the heart rate down.

Aerobic exercise, such as walking, bicycling, skating, swimming, or jogging, should be done for about 20–60 minutes most days per week. For optimal benefit, aerobic activity should be performed at a level that raises the heart rate to 60–85% of its maximum. Maximum heart rate is dependent on age and can be estimated by subtracting your age from 220. Therefore, a 20-year-old individual would have a maximum heart rate of 200 beats per minute and should exercise at a pace that keeps the heart rate between 120 and 170 beats per minute (Figure 8.2). A sedentary individual beginning an exercise program may find that mild exercise such as walking can raise the heart rate into this range. As fitness improves, you must perform more intense activity to elevate your heart rate to this level.

To improve and maintain flexibility, stretching exercises should be done at least three days a week. Muscles should be stretched to a position of mild discomfort and held for 10 to 30 seconds. Each stretch should be repeated three to five times.

Resistance training, such as weight lifting, should be done two to three days a week at the start of an exercise program, and two days a week after the desired strength has been achieved. This can be done with weights or with resistance-exercise machines. Each session should include a minimum of 8 to 10 exercises that train the major muscle groups. Each exercise should be repeated 8 to 12 times. The weights should be heavy enough to cause the muscle to be near exhaustion after the 8 to 12 repetitions. Increasing the amount of weight lifted will increase muscle strength, whereas increasing the number of repetitions will improve endurance.

How Much Should Children and Adolescents Exercise?

Children should spend about 60 minutes per day exercising, just like adults.[46] Activity for children should be developmentally appropriate and should include periods of moderate to vigorous activity lasting 10 to 15 minutes or more followed by periods of rest and recovery. Rather than a scheduled trip to the gym, children and adolescents should get their exercise by participating in fun activities with friends and family, such as playing tag, throwing a ball, or building a snow fort. Most American children do not get the recommended amount of exercise. This is because television, computers, and video games are often chosen over

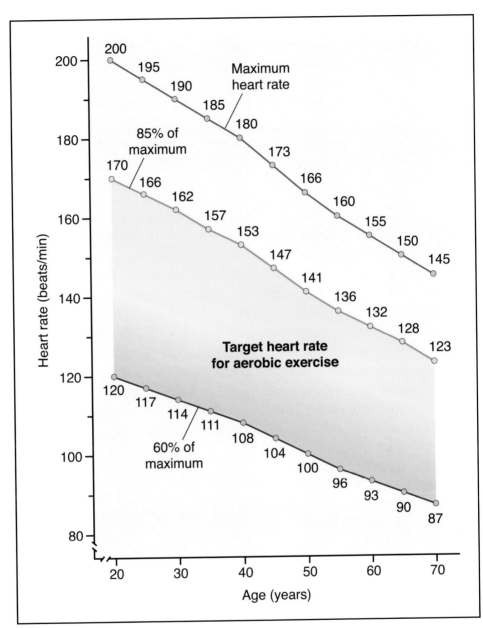

Figure 8.2 The target heart rate for aerobic exercise is 60–85% of a person's maximum heart rate, as can be seen on this graph. Maximum heart rate is estimated by subtracting an individual's age from 220. Exercise performed at this level will benefit cardiovascular fitness.

physical activity. Studies have found that children who watch four or more hours of television per day have more body fat and a greater body mass index (BMI) than those who spend fewer than two hours watching television.[47] Children who learn to enjoy physical activity are more likely to be active adults who maintain a healthy body weight and have a lower risk for disease. Learning by example is always best. Children who have physically active parents are the leanest and the fittest.

Getting Started

Finding a type of exercise that is enjoyable, a time to exercise that is realistic and convenient, and a place that is appropriate and safe are important first steps in adopting a pattern of increased activity. Some people prefer to exercise for a longer period once during the day while others may spread their exercise throughout the day in shorter, 10-minute-long bouts. The goal is an active lifestyle that can be continued over the long term.

Safety should be a concern in planning any exercise regimen. Before beginning, you should always check with a physician to be sure that your plans are safe, considering your medical history. Then the location and environment for exercise can be examined. Exercisers who use the street for walking or jogging should wear light-colored, reflective clothing so they can be seen by motorists. Weather conditions can be a health concern. Exercise should be reduced or curtailed in hot and humid conditions to avoid heat-related illness.

FACT BOX 8.2

Move Less—Gain More

Diet and lifestyle in the United States has had a great impact on body weight. In 1969, 4% of children between the ages of 6 and 11 were overweight. By 1999, that number had increased three-fold: 13% of children in this age group were overweight. Public health officials believe that this increase is related to a rise in calorie intake, combined with a reduction in physical activity among American youth.

In cooler environments, you need to wear clothing that allows for evaporation of sweat while also providing protection from the cold. Exercising with a partner is safer and often more enjoyable.

CONNECTIONS

A healthy lifestyle, including a nutritious diet and regular exercise, offers many health benefits, such as making it easier to maintain a proper body weight and keeping muscles, bones, and joints strong. It can help prevent or delay the onset of atherosclerosis, high blood pressure and stroke, diabetes, and cancer. A nutritious diet is one that provides the right number of calories to keep your weight within the desirable range; includes the proper balance of carbohydrates, protein, and fat choices; incorporates plenty of water; and has sufficient but not excessive amounts of essential vitamins and minerals. A healthy exercise program requires about an hour of moderate activity daily for adults as well as children and teens. A good exercise regimen should include aerobic exercise, strength training, and stretching exercises.

FACT BOX 8.3

Can Exercise Extend Your Life?

Medical research has found that the more you use your body, the longer it lasts. In a study of 17,000 Harvard alumni that examined mortality rates over a 22- to 26-year period, men who exercised lived longer than those who didn't. Moderate exercise was found to reduce the risk of heart disease and to raise life expectancy slightly. But to achieve a real shot at longevity, you have to work up a good sweat. Life expectancy was increased by two years in those who exercised strenuously for two or more hours a week.

By "strenuous," the researchers meant a continuous workout of at least 20 to 30 minutes that increased heart rate to 70–90% of the maximum. Strenuous activities include jogging, singles tennis, swimming, racquetball, biking, and aerobics classes. This amount of exercise was shown to reduce the risk of heart disease, hypertension, certain cancers, and diabetes; it also built cardiovascular fitness and lengthened life significantly.

Appendices

Appendix A

Dietary Reference Intake Values for Energy: Estimated Energy Requirement (EER) Equations and Values for Active Individuals by Life Stage Group

Life Stage Group	EER prediction equation	EER for Active Physical Activity Level (kcal/day)[a]	
		Male	**Female**
0 – 3 months	EER = (89 x weight of infant in kg – 100) + 175	538	493 (2 mo)[c]
4 – 6 months	EER = (89 x weight of infant in kg – 100) + 56	606	543 (5 mo)[c]
7 – 12 months	EER = (89 x weight of infant in kg – 100) + 22	743	676 (9 mo)[c]
1 – 2 years	EER = (89 x weight of infant in kg – 100) + 20	1046	992 (2 y)[c]
3 – 8 years			
male	EER = 88.5 – (61.9 x Age in yrs) + PA^b[(26.7 x Weight in kg) + (903 x Height in m)] + 20	1742 (6 y)[c]	
female	EER = 135.3 – (30.8 x Age in yrs) + PA^b[(10.0 x Weight in kg) + (934 x Height in m)] + 20		1642 (6 y)[c]
9 – 13 years			
male	EER = 88.5 – (61.9 x Age in yrs) + PA^b [(26.7 x Weight in kg) + (903 x Height in m)] + 25	2279 (11 y)[c]	
female	EER = 135.3 – (30.8 x Age in yrs) + PA^b [(10.0 x Weight in kg) + (934 x Height in m)] + 25		2071 (11 y)[c]
14 – 18 years			
male	EER = 88.5 – (61.9 x Age in yrs) + PA^b [(26.7 x Weight in kg) + (903 x Height in m)] + 25	3152 (16 y)[c]	
female	EER = 135.3 – (30.8 x Age in yrs) + PA^b [(10.0 x Weight in kg) + (934 x Height in m)] + 25		2368 (16 y)[c]
19 and older			
males	EER = 662 – (9.53 x Age in yrs) + PA^b[(15.91 x Weight in kg) + (539.6 x Height in m)]	3067 (19 y)[c]	
females	EER = 354 – (6.91 x Age in yrs) + PA^b[(9.36 x Weight in kg) + (726 x Height in m)]		2403 (19 y)[c]
Pregnancy			
14 –18 years			
1st trimester	Adolescent EER + 0		2368 (16 y)[c]
2nd trimester	Adolescent EER + 340 kcal		2708 (16 y)[c]
3rd trimester	Adolescent EER + 452 kcal		2820 (16 y)[c]
19 – 50 years			
1st trimester	Adult EER + 0		2403 (19 y)[c]
2nd trimester	Adult EER + 340 kcal		2743 (19 y)[c]
3rd trimester	Adult EER + 452 kcal		2855 (19 y)[c]
Lactation			
14 –18 years			
1st 6 mo	Adolescent EER + 330 kcal		2698 (16 y)[c]
2nd 6 mo	Adolescent EER + 400 kcal		2768 (16 y)[c]
19 – 50 years			
1st 6 mo	Adult EER + 330 kcal		2733 (19 y)[c]
2nd 6 mo	Adult EER + 400 kcal		2803 (19 y)[c]

[a] The intake that meets the average energy expenditure of individuals at a reference height, weight, and age
[b] See table entitled "PA Values" to determine the PA value for various ages, genders, and activity levels
[c] Value is calculated for an individual at the age in parentheses.

PA Values used to calculate EER

Physical Activity Level (PA)	Sedentary	Low active	Active	Very active
3 to 18 years				
Boys	1.00	1.13	1.26	1.42
Girls	1.00	1.16	1.31	1.56
≥ 19 years				
Men	1.00	1.11	1.25	1.48
Women	1.00	1.12	1.27	1.45

Source: Institute of Medicine, Food and Nutrition Board, "Dietary Reference Intakes for Energy, Carbohydrates, Fiber, Fat, Protein, and Amino Acids." Washington, D.C.: National Academy Press, 2002.

Acceptable Macronutrient Distribution Ranges (AMDR) for Healthy Diets as a Percent of Energy

Age	Carbohydrate	Added sugars	Total Fat	Linoleic acid	a-Linolenic acid	Protein
1-3 y	45-65	≤25	30-40	5-10	0.6-1.2	5-20
4-18 y	45-65	≤25	25-35	5-10	0.6-1.2	10-30
≥ 19 y	45-65	≤25	20-35	5-10	0.6-1.2	10-35

Source: Institute of Medicine, Food and Nutrition Board. "Dietary Reference Intakes for Energy, Carbohydrates, Fiber, Fat, Protein, and Amino Acids." Washington, D.C.: National Academy Press, 2002.

Dietary Reference Intakes: Recommended Intakes for Individuals: Carbohydrates, Fiber, Fat, Fatty Acids, and Protein

Life Stage Group	Carbohydrate (g/day)	Fiber (g/day)	Fat (g/day)	Linoleic acid (g/day)	a-Linolenic acid (g/day)	Protein (g/kg/day)	Protein (g/day)
Infants							
0-6 mo	60*	ND	31*	4.4*†	0.5*‡	1.52*	9.1*
7-12 mo	95*	ND	30*	4.6*†	0.5*‡	1.5	13.5
Children							
1-3 y	130	19*	ND	7*	0.7*	1.10	13
4-8 y	130	25*	ND	10*	0.9*	0.95	19
Males							
9-13 y	130	31*	ND	12*	1.2*	0.95	34
14-18 y	130	38*	ND	16*	1.6*	0.85	52
19-30 y	130	38*	ND	17*	1.6*	0.80	56
31-50 y	130	38*	ND	17*	1.6*	0.80	56
51-70 y	130	30*	ND	14*	1.6*	0.80	56
> 70 y	130	30*	ND	14*	1.6*	0.80	56
Females							
9-13 y	130	26*	ND	10*	1.0*	0.95	34
14-18 y	130	26*	ND	11*	1.1*	0.85	46
19-30 y	130	25*	ND	12*	1.1*	0.80	46
31-50 y	130	25*	ND	12*	1.1*	0.80	46
51-70 y	130	21*	ND	11*	1.1*	0.80	46
> 70 y	130	21*	ND	11*	1.1*	0.80	46
Pregnancy	175	28*	ND	13*	1.4*	1.1	RDA+25g
Lactation	210	29*	ND	13*	1.3*	1.1	RDA+25g

ND = not determined
* Values are AI (Adequate intakes)
† Refers to all n-6 polyunsaturated fatty acids
‡ Refers to all n-3 polyunsaturated fatty acids

Source: Institute of Medicine, Food and Nutrition Board. "Dietary Reference Intakes for Energy, Carbohydrates, Fiber, Fat, Protein, and Amino Acids." Washington, D.C.: National Academy Press, 2002.

Appendix B

Dietary Reference Intakes: Recommended Intakes for Individuals: Vitamins

Life Stage Group	Vitamin A (µg/day)[a]	Vitamin C (mg/day)	Vitamin D (µg/day)[b,c]	Vitamin E (mg/day)[d]	Vitamin K (µg/day)	Thiamin (mg/day)	Riboflavin (mg/day)	Niacin (mg/day)[e]	Vitamin B_6 (mg/day)	Folate (µg/day)[f]	Vitamin B_{12} (µg/day)	Pantothenic Acid (mg/day)	Biotin (µg/day)	Choline[g] (mg/day)
Infants														
0-6 mo	400*	40*	5*	4*	2.0*	0.2*	0.3*	2*	0.1*	65*	0.4*	1.7*	5*	125*
7-12 mo	500*	50*	5*	5*	2.5*	0.3*	0.4*	4*	0.3*	80*	0.5*	1.8*	6*	150*
Children														
1-3 y	300	15	5*	6	30*	0.5	0.5	6	0.5	150	0.9	2*	8*	200*
4-8 y	400	25	5*	7	55*	0.6	0.6	8	0.5	200	1.2	3*	12*	250*
Males														
9-13 y	600	45	5*	11	60*	0.9	0.9	12	1.0	300	1.8	4*	20*	315*
14-18 y	900	75	5*	15	75*	1.2	1.3	16	1.3	400	2.4	5*	25*	550*
19-30 y	900	90	5*	15	120*	1.2	1.3	16	1.3	400	2.4	5*	30*	550*
31-50 y	900	90	5*	15	120*	1.2	1.3	16	1.3	400	2.4	5*	30*	550*
51-70 y	900	90	10*	15	120*	1.2	1.3	16	1.7	400	2.4[h]	5*	30*	550*
> 70 y	900	90	15*	15	120*	1.2	1.3	16	1.7	400	2.4[h]	5*	30*	550*
Females														
9-13 y	600	45	5*	11	60*	0.9	0.9	12	1.0	300	1.8	4*	20*	375*
14-18 y	700	65	5*	15	75*	1.0	1.0	14	1.2	400[i]	2.4	5*	25*	400*
19-30 y	700	75	5*	15	90*	1.1	1.1	14	1.3	400[i]	2.4	5*	30*	425*
31-50 y	700	75	5*	15	90*	1.1	1.1	14	1.3	400[i]	2.4	5*	30*	425*
51-70 y	700	75	10*	15	90*	1.1	1.1	14	1.5	400	2.4[h]	5*	30*	425*
> 70 y	700	75	15*	15	90*	1.1	1.1	14	1.5	400	2.4[h]	5*	30*	425*
Pregnancy														
≤ 18 y	750	80	5*	15	75*	1.4	1.4	18	1.9	600[j]	2.6	6*	30*	450*
14-18 y	770	85	5*	15	90*	1.4	1.4	18	1.9	600[j]	2.6	6*	30*	450*
19-30 y	770	85	5*	15	90*	1.4	1.4	18	1.9	600[j]	2.6	6*	30*	450*
Lactation														
≤ 18 y	1200	115	5*	19	75*	1.4	1.6	17	2.0	500	2.8	7*	35*	550*
14-18 y	1300	120	5*	19	90*	1.4	1.6	17	2.0	500	2.8	7*	35*	550*
19-30 y	1300	120	5*	19	90*	1.4	1.6	17	2.0	500	2.8	7*	35*	550*

NOTE: This table (taken from the DRI reports, see www.nap.edu) presents Recommended Dietary Allowances (RDAs) in **bold** type and Adequate Intakes (AIs) in ordinary type followed by an asterisk (*). RDAs and AIs may both be used as goals for individual intakes. RDAs are set up to meet the needs of almost all (97–98%) individuals in a group. For healthy breastfed infants, the AI is the mean intake. The AI for all other life stage and gender groups is believed to cover needs of all individuals in the group, but lack of data or uncertainty in the data prevent being able to specify with confidence the percentage of individuals covered by this intake.

[a] As retinol activity equivalents (RAEs). 1 RAE = 1 µg retinol, 12 µg β-carotene, 24 µg β-carotene, or 24 µg β-cryptoxanthin in foods. To calculate RAEs from REs of provitamin A carotenoids in foods, divide RE by 2. For preformed vitamin A in foods or supplements and for provitamin A carotenoids in supplements, 1 RE = 1 RAE.

[b] Cholecalciferol. 1 µg cholecalciferol = 40 IU vitamin D.

[c] In the absence of exposure to adequate sunlight.

[d] As α-tocopherol, which includes RRR-α-tocopherol, the only form of α-tocopherol that occurs naturally in foods, and the 2R-stereoisomeric forms of α-tocopherol (RRR-, RSR-, RRS-, and RSS-α-tocopherol). Does not include the 2S-stereoisomeric forms of α-tocopherol (SRR-, SSR-, SRS-, and SSS- α -tocopherol), also found in food and supplements.

[e] As niacin equivalents (NEs), 1mg niacin = 60 mg tryptophan; 0-6 months = preformed niacin (not NE).

[f] As dietary folate equivalents (DFEs. 1 DFE = 1 µg food folate = 0.6 µg folic acid from fortified food or as a supplement consumed with food = 0.5 µg of a supplement taken on an empty stomach.

[g] Although AIs have been set for choline, there are few data to assess whether a dietary supplement of choline is needed at all stages of the lifecycle, and it may be that the choline requirement can be met by endogenous synthesis at some of these stages.

[h] Because 10-30% of older people may malabsorb food-bound B_{12}, it is advisable for those older than 50 years to meet their RFD mainly by consuming foods fortified with B_{12} or containing B_{12}.

[i] In view of evidence linking folate intake with neural tube defects in the fetus, it is recommended that all women capable of becoming pregnant consume 400 µg from supplements or fortified foods in addition to intake of food folate from a varied diet.

[j] It is assumed that women will consume 400 µg from supplements or fortified foods until their pregnancy is confirmed and they enter prenatal care, which ordinarily occurs after the end of the periconceptional period – the critical time for neural tube formation.

Source: Trumbo, P., A. Yates, S. Schlicker, M. Poos. "Dietary Reference Intakes: Vitamin A, Vitamin K, Arsenic, Boron, Chrominm, Copper, Iodine, Iron, Manganese, Molybdenum, Nickel, Silicon, Vanadium, and Zinc." *Journal of the American Dietetic Association* 101, no. 3 (2001) 294-301.

Dietary Reference Intakes: Recommended Intakes for Individuals: Minerals

Life Stage Group	Calcium (mg/day)	Chromium (µg/day)	Copper (µg/day)	Fluoride (mg/day)	Iodine (µg/day)	Iron (mg/day)	Magnesium (mg/day)	Manganese (mg/day)	Molybdenum (µg/day)	Phosphorus (mg/day)	Selenium (µg/day)	Zinc (mg/day)
Infants												
0-6 mo	210*	0.2*	200*	0.01*	110*	0.27*	30*	0.003*	2*	100*	15*	2*
7-12 mo	270*	5.5*	220*	0.5*	130*	11	75*	0.6*	3*	275*	20*	3
Children												
1-3 y	500*	11*	340	0.7*	90	7	80	1.2*	17	460	20	3
4-8 y	800*	15*	440	1*	90	10	130	1.5*	22	500	30	5
Males												
9-13 y	1,300*	25*	700	2*	120	8	240	1.9*	34	1,250	40	8
14-18 y	1,300*	35*	890	3*	150	11	410	2.2*	43	1,250	55	11
19-30 y	1,000*	35*	900	4*	150	8	400	2.3*	45	700	55	11
31-50 y	1,000*	35*	900	4*	150	8	420	2.3*	45	700	55	11
51-70 y	1,200*	30*	900	4*	150	8	420	2.3*	45	700	55	11
>70 y	1,200*	30*	900	4*	150	8	420	2.3*	45	700	55	11
Females												
9-13 y	1,300*	21*	700	2*	120	8	240	1.6*	34	1,250	40	8
14-18 y	1,300*	24*	890	3*	150	15	360	1.6*	43	1,250	55	9
19-30 y	1,000*	25*	900	3*	150	18	310	1.8*	45	700	55	8
31-50 y	1,000*	25*	900	3*	150	18	320	1.8*	45	700	55	8
51-70 y	1,200*	20*	900	3*	150	8	320	1.8*	45	700	55	8
>70 y	1,200*	20*	900	3*	150	8	320	1.8*	45	700	55	8
Pregnancy												
≤18 y	1,300*	29*	1,000	3*	220	27	400	2.0*	50	1,250	60	13
14-18 y	1,000*	30*	1,000	3*	220	27	350	2.0*	50	700	60	11
19-30 y	1,000*	30*	1,000	3*	220	27	360	2.0*	50	700	60	11
Lactation												
≤18 y	1,300*	44*	1,300	3*	290	10	360	2.6*	50	1,250	70	14
14-18 y	1,300*	45*	1,300	3*	290	9	310	2.6*	50	700	70	12
19-30 y	1,300*	45*	1,300	3*	290	9	320	2.6*	50	700	70	12

NOTE: This table (taken from the DRI reports, see www.nap.edu) presents Recommended Dietary Allowances (RDAs) in **bold** type and Adequate Intakes (AIs) in ordinary type followed by an asterisk (*). RDAs and AIs may both be used as goals for individual intakes. RDAs are set up to meet the needs of almost all (97-98%) individuals in a group. For healthy breastfed infants, the AI is the mean intake. The AI for all other life stage and gender groups is believed to cover needs of all individuals in the group, but lack of data or uncertainty in the data prevents being able to specify with confidence the percentage of individuals covered by this intake.

Dietary Reference Intakes (DRIs): Tolerable Upper Intake Levels (UL[a]): Vitamins

Life Stage Group	Vitamin A (µg/day)[b]	Vitamin C (mg/day)	Vitamin D (µg/day)	Vitamin E (mg/day)[c,d]	Vitamin K	Thiamin	Riboflavin	Niacin (mg/day)[d]	Vitamin B6 (mg/day)	Folate (µg/day)[d]	Vitamin B12	Pantothenic Acid	Biotin	Choline (mg/day)	Carotenoids[e]
Infants															
0-6 mo	600	ND[f]	25	ND[f]	ND	ND	ND	ND	ND	ND	ND	ND	ND	ND	ND
7-12 mo	600	ND	25	ND	ND	ND	ND	ND	ND	ND	ND	ND	ND	ND	ND
Children															
1-3 y	600	400	50	200	ND	ND	ND	10	30	300	ND	ND	ND	1.0	ND
4-8 y	900	650	50	300	ND	ND	ND	15	40	400	ND	ND	ND	1.0	ND
Males, Females															
9-13 y	1,700	1,200	50	600	ND	ND	ND	20	60	600	ND	ND	ND	2.0	ND
14-18 y	2,800	1,800	50	800	ND	ND	ND	30	80	800	ND	ND	ND	3.0	ND
19-70 y	3,000	2,000	50	1,000	ND	ND	ND	35	100	1,000	ND	ND	ND	3.5	ND
>70 y	3,000	2,000	50	1,000	ND	ND	ND	35	100	1,000	ND	ND	ND	3.5	ND
Pregnancy															
≤18 y	2,800	1,800	50	800	ND	ND	ND	30	80	800	ND	ND	ND	3.0	ND
19-50 y	3,000	2,000	50	1,000	ND	ND	ND	35	100	1,000	ND	ND	ND	3.5	ND
Lactation															
≤18 y	2,800	1,800	50	800	ND	ND	ND	30	80	800	ND	ND	ND	3.0	ND
19-50 y	3,000	2,000	50	1,000	ND	ND	ND	35	100	1,000	ND	ND	ND	3.5	ND

[a]UL = The maximum level of daily nutrient intake that is likely to pose no risk of adverse effects. Unless otherwise specified, the UL represents total intake from food, water, and supplements. Due to lack of suitable data, ULs could not be established for vitamin K, thiamin, riboflavin, vitamin B12, pantothenic acid, biotin, or carotenoids. In the absence of ULs, extra caution may be warranted in consuming levels above recommended intakes.

[b]As preformed vitamin A only.

[c]As α-tocopherol; applies to any for of supplemental α-tocopherol.

[d]The ULs for vitamin E, niacin, and folate apply to synthetic forms obtained from supplements, fortified foods, or a combination of the two.

[e]β-Carotene supplements are advised only to serve as a provitamin A source for individuals at risk of vitamin A deficiency.

[f]ND=Not determinable due to lack of data of adverse effects in this age group and concern with regard to lack of ability to handle excess amounts. Source of intakes should be from food only to prevent high levels of intake.

Dietary Reference Intakes (DRIs): Tolerable Upper Intake Levels (UL[a]): Minerals

Life Stage Group	Arsenic[b]	Boron (mg/day)	Calcium (g/day)	Chromium	Copper (μg/day)	Fluoride (mg/day)	Iodine (μg/day)	Iron (mg/day)	Magnesium (mg/day)[c]	Manganese (mg/day)	Molybdenum (μg/day)	Nickel (mg/day)	Phosphorus (g/day)	Selenium (μg/day)	Silicon[d]	Vanadium (mg/day)[e]	Zinc (mg/day)
Infants																	
0-6 mo	ND[f]	ND	ND	ND	ND	0.7	ND	40	ND	ND	ND	ND	ND	45	ND	ND	4
7-12 mo	ND	ND	ND	ND	ND	0.9	ND	40	ND	ND	ND	ND	ND	60	ND	ND	5
Children																	
1-3 y	ND	3	2.5	ND	1,000	1.3	200	40	65	2	300	0.2	3	90	ND	ND	7
4-8 y	ND	6	2.5	ND	3,000	2.2	300	40	110	3	600	0.3	3	150	ND	ND	12
Males, Females																	
9-13 y	ND	11	2.5	ND	5,000	10	600	40	350	6	1,100	0.6	4	280	ND	ND	23
14-18 y	ND	17	2.5	ND	8,000	10	900	45	350	9	1,700	1.0	4	400	ND	ND	34
19-70 y	ND	20	2.5	ND	10,000	10	1,100	45	350	11	2,000	1.0	4	400	ND	1.8	40
>70 y	ND	20	2.5	ND	10,000	10	1,100	45	350	11	2,000	1.0	3	400	ND	1.8	40
Pregnancy																	
≤18 y	ND	17	2.5	ND	8,000	10	900	45	350	9	1,700	1.0	3.5	400	ND	ND	34
19-50 y	ND	20	2.5	ND	10,000	10	1,100	45	350	11	2,000	1.0	3.5	400	ND	ND	40
Lactation																	
≤18 y	ND	17	2.5	ND	8,000	10	900	45	350	9	1,700	1.0	4	400	ND	ND	34
19-50 y	ND	20	2.5	ND	10,000	10	1,100	45	350	11	2,000	1.0	4	400	ND	ND	40

[a]UL= the maximum level of daily nutrient intake that is likely to pose no risk of adverse effects. Unless otherwise specified, the UL represents total intake from food, water, and supplements. Due to lack of suitable data, ULs could not be established for arsenic, chromium, and silicon. In the absence of ULs, extra caution may be warranted in consuming levels above recommended intakes.

[b]Although the UL was not determined for arsenic, there is no justification for adding arsenic to food or supplements.

[c]The ULs for magnesium represent intake from a pharmacological agent only and do not include intake from food and water.

[d]Although silicon has not been shown to cause adverse effects in humans, there is no justification for adding silicon to supplements.

[e]Although vanadium in food has not been shown to cause adverse effects in humans, there is no justification for adding vanadium to food and vanadium supplements should be used with caution. The UL is based on adverse effects in laboratory animals and this data could be used to set a UL for adults from not children and adolescents. Source of intake should be from food only to prevent high levels of intake.

[f]ND=Not determinable due to lack of data of adverse effects in this age group and concern with regard to lack of ability to handle excess amounts.

Appendix B

Dietary Reference Intakes: Recommended Intakes and Tolerable Upper Intake Levels (UL): Water, Potassium, Sodium, and Chloride						
Life Stage Group	**Water** [a] (liters)	**Potassium** [a,b] (mg)	**Sodium** (mg)		**Chloride** (mg)	
			Recommended Intake	UL	Recommended Intake	UL
Infants						
0–6 mo	0.7	0.4	0.12	-	0.18	-
7–12 mo	0.8	0.7	0.37	-	0.58	-
Children						
1–3 y	1.3	3.0	1.0	1.5	1.5	2.3
4–8 y	1.7	3.8	1.2	1.9	1.9	2.9
Males						
9–13 y	2.4	4.5	1.5	2.2	2.3	3.4
14–18 y	3.3	4.7	1.5	2.3	2.3	3.6
19–30 y	3.7	4.7	1.5	2.3	2.3	3.6
31–50 y	3.7	4.7	1.5	2.3	2.3	3.6
51–70 y	3.7	4.7	1.3	2.3	2.0	3.6
>70 y	3.7	4.7	1.2	2.3	1.8	3.6
Females						
9–13 y	2.1	4.5	1.5	2.2	2.3	3.4
14–18 y	2.3	4.7	1.5	2.3	2.3	3.6
19–30 y	2.7	4.7	1.5	2.3	2.3	3.6
31–50 y	2.7	4.7	1.5	2.3	2.3	3.6
51–70 y	2.7	4.7	1.3	2.3	2.0	3.6
>70 y	2.7	4.7	1.2	2.3	1.8	3.6

[a] No UL has been established for water or potassium.

[b] The recommended intake is the same for all groups over 14 years except lactating women, which is 5.1 mg

CDC Growth Charts: United States

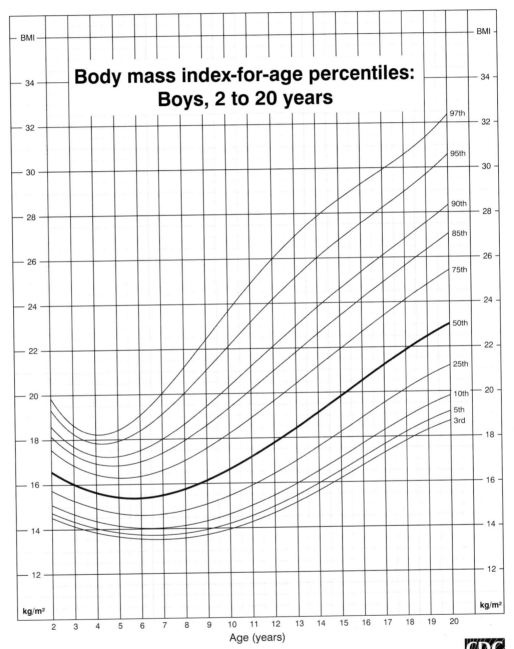

Body mass index-for-age percentiles: Boys, 2 to 20 years

Age (years)

Published May 30, 2000.
SOURCE: Developed by the National Center for Health Statistics in collaboration with
the National Center for Chronic Disease Prevention and Health Promotion (2000).

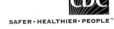

SAFER · HEALTHIER · PEOPLE™

CDC Growth Charts: United States

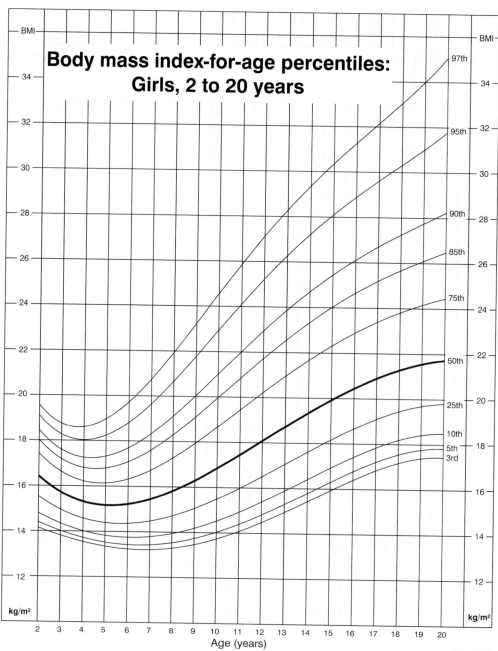

Body mass index-for-age percentiles:
Girls, 2 to 20 years

Age (years)

Published May 30, 2000.
SOURCE: Developed by the National Center for Health Statistics in collaboration with
the National Center for Chronic Disease Prevention and Health Promotion (2000).

CDC
SAFER·HEALTHIER·PEOPLE™

Glossary

Acetyl CoA An intermediate formed during the breakdown of carbohydrates, fatty acids, and amino acids. It consists of a 2-carbon compound attached to a molecule of CoA.

Actin The contractile protein that makes up the thin filaments in muscle fibers.

Adequate Intakes (AIs) DRI values used as a goal for intake when there is insufficient evidence to establish an RDA.

Adipose tissue Tissue found under the skin and around body organs that is composed of fat-storing cells.

Aerobic capacity (also called **maximum oxygen consumption** and **VO$_2$max**) A person's maximum capacity to generate ATP by aerobic metabolism. It depends on the amount of oxygen that can be delivered to and used by the muscle.

Aerobic exercise Activity that uses aerobic metabolism and improves cardiovascular fitness.

Aerobic metabolism Metabolism requiring oxygen. The complete breakdown of glucose, fatty acids, and amino acids to carbon dioxide and water occurs only via aerobic metabolism.

Aldosterone A hormone that increases sodium reabsorption and therefore enhances water retention by the kidney.

Amenorrhea Absence or abnormal cessation of menstrual periods in women.

Amino acids Nitrogen-containing organic compounds that function as the building blocks of protein.

Anabolic steroids Synthetic fat-soluble hormones used by some athletes to increase muscle mass.

Anaerobic metabolism The processing of ATP from glucose in the muscles in the absence of oxygen; also called anaerobic glycolysis.

Angiotensin II A compound that causes blood vessel walls to constrict and stimulates the release of the hormone aldosterone.

Anorexia nervosa An eating disorder that is characterized by a distorted body image, self-starvation, and loss of 15% or more of body weight.

Antidiuretic hormone (ADH) A hormone secreted by the pituitary gland that increases the amount of water reabsorbed by the kidney and therefore retained in the body.

Antioxidant A substance that is able to neutralize reactive molecules and hence reduce the amount of oxidative damage that occurs.

Apparent temperature or **heat index** A measure of how hot it feels when the relative humidity is added to the actual temperature.

ATP (adenosine triphosphate) The high-energy molecule used by the body to perform energy-requiring activities.

Atrophy A wasting away or decrease in size of a body part due to an abnormality, poor nutrition, or lack of use.

Beta-hydroxy-beta-methylbutyrate (HMB) A compound generated from the breakdown of the amino acid leucine that is used by athletes as an ergogenic aid to reduce the muscle damage associated with intense physical effort.

Beta-oxidation The breakdown of fatty acids into 2-carbon units that form acetyl CoA.

Bicarbonate A compound present in the body that prevents changes in acidity. It is used as an ergogenic aid to neutralize lactic acid.

Bulimia nervosa An eating disorder characterized by a cycle of binging and purging.

Calories (Kilocalories) Units of heat that express the amount of energy provided by foods.

Carbohydrate loading or **glycogen supercompensation** A regimen of diet and exercise that is designed to load muscle glycogen stores beyond their normal capacity.

Cardiac muscle The type of muscle tissue that makes up the heart.

Cardiac output The amount of blood pumped by the heart during a one-minute period.

Carnitine A compound made from the amino acids lysine and methionine that is needed to transport fatty acids into the mitochondria. It is used as an ergogenic aid.

Glossary

Cellular respiration The reactions that break down glucose, fatty acids, and amino acids in the presence of oxygen to produce carbon dioxide, water, and energy in the form of ATP.

Cholesterol A lipid made only by animal cells that consists of multiple chemical rings.

Chromium picolinate A dietary supplement sold as an ergogenic aid that claims to increase lean body mass and decrease body fat.

Citric acid cycle Also known as the Krebs cycle or the tricarboxylic acid cycle, this is the stage of respiration in which acetyl CoA is broken down into two molecules of carbon dioxide.

Creatine A nitrogen-containing compound found in muscle, where it is used to make creatine phosphate. It is used as an ergogenic aid to increase short-duration, high-power performance and increase muscle mass.

Creatine phosphate A high-energy compound found in muscle that can be broken down to form ATP.

Dehydration A reduction in the amount of body water.

Dietary References Intakes (DRIs) A set of four reference values for the intake of nutrients and food components that can be used for planning and assessing the diets of healthy people in the United States and Canada.

Electrolytes Substances that separate in water to form positively and negatively charged ions. In nutrition, this term refers to sodium, potassium, and chloride.

Electron transport chain The final stage of cellular respiration in which electrons are passed down a chain of molecules to oxygen, forming water and producing ATP.

Enzyme Protein molecules in the body that accelerate the rate of chemical reactions in the body but are not altered by the process.

Ephedra A naturally occurring substance derived from the Chinese herb *Ma huang*. It acts as a stimulant, increasing blood pressure and heart rate.

Ergogenic aids Substances that can enhance athletic performance.

Erythropoietin (EPO) A peptide hormone that stimulates stem cells in the bone marrow to differentiate into red blood cells. It is used as an ergogenic aid to increase endurance.

Estimated Average Requirements (EARs) Intakes that meet the estimated nutrient needs (as defined by a specific indicator of adequacy) of 50% of individuals in a gender and life-stage group.

Estimated Energy Requirements (EERs) Recommendations for energy needs that are based on the amount of energy predicted to maintain energy balance in a healthy person of a defined age, gender, height, weight, and level of physical activity.

Extracellular fluid The fluid located outside cells. It includes fluid found in the blood, lymph, gastrointestinal tract, spinal column, eyes, and joints, and that found between cells and tissues.

Fast twitch muscle fibers Muscle cells that can contract very quickly and have a great capacity for ATP production via anaerobic metabolism.

Fatigue The inability to continue an activity at an optimal level.

Fatty acids Lipids made up of chains of carbons linked to hydrogens with an acid group at one end.

Female athlete triad A syndrome in young female athletes that involves disordered eating, amenorrhea, and low bone density.

Fiber Substances in food that cannot be broken down by human digestive enzymes.

Free radicals Groups of atoms with one or more unpaired electrons; they are often created inside the body as the result of outside pollutants (such as smoke) and can cause severe damage to body cells.

Ginseng An herbal supplement promoted to increase endurance.

Gluconeogenesis The synthesis of glucose from simple noncarbohydrate molecules. Amino acids from protein are the primary source of carbons for glucose synthesis.

Glucose A monosaccharide that is the primary form of carbohydrate used to produce energy in the body.

Glossary

Glycogen A carbohydrate made of many glucose molecules linked together in a highly branched structure. It is the storage form of carbohydrate in animals.

Glycolysis A metabolic pathway in the cytoplasm of the cell that splits glucose into two 3-carbon molecules. The energy released from one molecule of glucose is used to make two ATP molecules.

Growth hormone A peptide hormone produced by the pituitary gland that is important for growth and maintenance of lean tissue.

Homeostasis A physiological state in which a stable internal environment is maintained.

Hormone A chemical messenger that is secreted into the blood by one tissue and acts on cells in another part of the body.

Hypertrophy Enlargement or overgrowth of tissue.

Hyponatremia A low concentration of sodium in the blood.

Insensible losses Fluid losses that are not perceived by the senses, such as evaporation of water through the skin and respiratory tract.

Interstitial fluid The portion of the extracellular fluid located in the spaces between cells.

Intracellular fluid The fluid located inside cells.

Ketones Molecules formed when there is not sufficient carbohydrate to completely metabolize the acetyl CoA produced from fat breakdown.

Kilocalorie See **Calorie**.

Kilojoule A measure of work that can be used to express energy intake and energy output; 4.18 kjoules = 1 kcalorie.

Lactic acid An acid produced as an end product of anaerobic metabolism.

Malnutrition Any condition resulting from an energy or nutrient intake either above or below that which is optimal.

Maximal oxygen consumption See **Aerobic capacity**.

Medium chain triglycerides (MCTs) Fats containing fatty acids that have 8 to 10 carbons in their carbon chain. These fatty acids can be absorbed directly into the blood and do not require carnitine for transport into the mitochondria.

Metabolism The sum of all the chemical reactions that take place within a living organism.

Myofibril Rodlike structures inside muscle cells that are responsible for muscle contraction.

Myosin The contractile protein that makes up the thick filaments of muscle fibers.

Nutrients Chemical substances in foods that provide energy, structure, and regulation for body processes.

Nutrition A science that studies the interactions that occur between living organisms and food.

Osmosis The movement of water across a membrane in a direction that will equalize the concentration of dissolved substances on each side.

Osteoporosis A bone disorder characterized by a reduction in bone mass, increased bone fragility, and an increased risk of fractures.

Overnutrition Poor nutritional status resulting from a dietary intake in excess of that which is optimal for health.

Overtraining syndrome A collection of emotional, behavioral, and physical symptoms caused by repeatedly training without sufficient rest to allow for recovery.

Phytochemical A substance found in plant foods that is not an essential nutrient but may have health-promoting properties.

Pyruvate A 3-carbon molecule produced when glucose is broken down by glycolysis.

Recommended Dietary Allowances (RDAs) A recommended intake that is sufficient to meet the nutrient needs of almost all healthy people in a specific life-stage and gender group.

Renin An enzyme released by the kidneys when blood pressure drops that aids in the production of angiotensin II.

Glossary

Ribose A sugar that is needed to synthesize RNA and ATP.

Saturated fats Triglycerides containing fatty acids with no carbon-carbon double bonds.

Skeletal muscles Muscles attached to the skeleton that are under voluntary control.

Slow twitch muscle fibers Muscle cells that can continue to contract for long periods and rely primarily on aerobic metabolism.

Smooth muscle A type of muscle that is not under voluntary control. It lines blood vessels, air passageways, and the walls of glands and other organs.

Starch A carbohydrate made of many glucose molecules linked in straight or branching chains. The bonds that hold the glucose molecules together can be broken by the human digestive enzymes.

Stroke volume The amount of blood pumped by the heart with each beat.

Sugars The simplest form of carbohydrate.

Tolerable Upper Intake Level (UL) The maximum daily intake by an individual that is unlikely to pose risks of adverse health effects to almost all individuals in the specified life-stage and gender group.

Triglycerides A fat composed of three fatty acids and a molecule of glycerol.

Unsaturated fats Triglycerides containing fatty acids with one or more carbon-carbon double bonds.

Urea A nitrogen-containing waste product that is excreted in the urine.

VO_2max See **Aerobic capacity**.

1. Institute of Medicine, Food and Nutrition Board. "Dietary Reference Intakes for Energy, Carbohydrates, Fiber, Fat, Protein, and Amino Acids." Washington, D.C.: National Academy Press, 2002.

2. Manore, M., and Thompson, J. *Sport Nutrition for Health and Performance*. Champaign, IL: Human Kinetics, 2000.

3. McArdle, W.D., Katch, F.I., and Katch, V.L. *Exercise Physiology: Energy, Nutrition, and Human Performance*, 5th ed. Baltimore: Lippincott Williams & Wilkens, 2001.

4. Rhoades, R., and Pflanzer, R. *Human Physiology*, 3rd ed. Philadelphia: Saunders College Publishing, 1996.

5. Freudenrich, Craig C. "How Exercise Works: Getting the Most from Muscles." Available online at *http://entertainment.howstuffworks.com/sports-physiology6.htm*.

6. Quinn, Elizabeth. "Fast and Slow Twitch Muscle Fibers: How They Affect Your Performance." Available online at *http://sportsmedicine.about.com/library/weekly/aa080901a.htm*.

7. JADA. "Nutrition and Athletic Performance—Position of the American Dietetic Association, Dietitians of Canada, and American College of Sports Medicine." *Journal of the American Dietetic Association* 100 (2000): 1543–1556.

8. McArdle, Katch, and Katch, p. 578.

9. Askew, E.W. "Nutrition and performance in hot, cold, and high-altitude environments." *Nutrition in Exercise and Sport*, 3rd ed., ed. I. Wolinsky. Boca Raton: CRC Press, 1998, pp. 597–619.

10. Shen, H-P. "Body fluids and water balance." *Biochemical and Physiological Aspects of Human Nutrition*, ed. M. Stipanuk. Philadelphia: W. B. Saunders, 2000, pp. 843–865.

11. Institute of Medicine, Food and Nutrition Board. "Dietary Reference Intakes for Water, Potassium, Sodium, Chloride, and Sulfate." Washington, D.C.: National Academy Press, 2004.

12. "Salt and the Ultraendurance athlete." Available online at *http://www.rice.edu/~jenky/sports/salt.html*.

13. Senay, L.C. "Water and electrolytes during physical activity," *Nutrition in Exercise and Sport*, 3rd ed., ed. I. Wolinski. Boca Raton: CRC Press, 1998, pp. 257–276.

14. Dekkers, J.C., van Doornen, L.J.P., and Kemper, H.C.G. "The role of antioxidant vitamins and enzymes in the prevention of exercise-induced muscle damage." *Sports Medicine* 21 (1996): 213–238.

15. Lukaski, H.C. "Chromium as a supplement." *Annual Review of Nutrition* 19 (1999): 279–301.

16. Stearns, D.M., Wise, J.P., Patierno, S.R., and Wetterhahn, K.E. "Chromium (III) picolinate produces damage in Chinese hamster ovary cells." *Federation of American Societies for Experimental Biology Journal* 9 (1995): 1643–1648.

17. Kato, I., Vogelman, J.H., Dilman, V., et al. "Effect of supplementation with chromium picolinate on antibody titers to 5-hydroxymethyl uracil." *European Journal of Epidemiology* 14 (1998): 621–626.

18. Williams, M.H. "Facts and fallacies of purported ergogenic amino acid supplements." *Clinical Sports Medicine* 18 (1999): 633–649.

References

19. McArdle, Katch, and Katch, p. 561.

20. Van Hall, G., Saris, W.H., van de Schoor, P.A., and Wagenmakers, A.J. "The effect of free glutamine and peptide ingestion on the rate of muscle glycogen resynthesis in man." *International Journal of Sports Medicine.* 21 (2000): 25–30.

21. Davis, J.M., Welsh, R.S., De Volve, K.L., and Alderson, N.A. "Effects of branched-chain amino acids and carbohydrate on fatigue during intermittent, high-intensity running." *International Journal of Sports Medicine* 20 (1999): 309–314.

22. Brass, E.P. "Supplemental carnitine and exercise." *American Journal of Clinical Nutrition* 72 (supplement) (2000): 618S–623S.

23. Misell, L.M., Lagomarcino, N.D., Schuster, V., and Kern, M. "Chronic medium-chain triacylglycerol consumption and endurance performance in trained runners." *Journal of Sports Medicine and Physical Fitness* 41(2) (2001): 210–215.

24. Horowitz, J.F., Mora-Rodriguez, R., Byerley, L.O., and Coyle, E.F. "Preexercise medium-chain triglyceride ingestion does not alter muscle glycogen use during exercise." *Journal of Applied Physiology* 88(1) (2000): 219–225.

25. Terjung, R.L., Clarkson, P., Eichner, E.R., et al. "American College of Sports Medicine roundtable: The physiological and health effects of oral creatine supplementation." *Medicine and Science in Sports and Exercise* 32 (2000): 706–717.

26. Feldman, E.B. "Creatine: a dietary supplement and ergogenic aid." *Nutrition Reviews* 57 (1999): 45–50.

27. Dempsey, R.L., Mazzone, M.F., and Meurer, L.N. "Does oral creatine supplementation improve strength? A meta-analysis." *Journal of Family Practice* 1(11) (2001): 945–951.

28. Poortmans, J.R., and Francaux, M. "Adverse effects of creatine supplementation: fact or fiction?" *Sports Medicine* 30 (2000): 155–170.

29. Spriet, L.L. "Caffeine and performance." *International Journal of Sport Nutrition* 5 (supplement) (1995): 84S–99S.

30. Kreider, R.B., Melton, C., Greenwood, M., et al. "Effects of oral d-ribose supplementation on anaerobic capacity and selected metabolic markers in healthy males." *International Journal of Sport Nutrition and Exercise Metabolism* 13 (1) (2003): 87–96.

31. Op't Eijnde, B., Van Leemputte, M., Brouns, F., et al. "No effects of oral ribose supplementation on repeated maximal exercise and de novo ATP resynthesis." *Journal of Applied Physiology* 91(5) (2002): 2275–2281.

32. McArdle, Katch, and Katch, pp. 570–571.

33. Bucci, L.R. "Selected herbals and human exercise performance." *American Journal of Clinical Nutrition* 72 (2000): 624S–636S.

34. U.S. Food and Drug Administration. Evidence Report/Technology Assessment Number 76. "Ephedra and Ephedrine for Weight Loss and Athletic Performance Enhancement: Clinical Efficacy and Side Effects." Available online at *http://www.fda.gov/bbs/topics/ NEWS/ephedra/summary.html.*

35. Bent, S., Tiedt, T.N., Odden, M.C., and Shlipak, M.G. "The relative safety of ephedra compared with other herbal products." *Annals of Internal Medicine* 138 (2003): 468–471.

36. U.S. Food and Drug Administration. FDA White Paper, Health Effects of Androsteinedione, March 11, 2004. Available online at *http://www.fda.gov/oc/whitepapers/andro.html.*

37. Ritter, S.K. "Faster, higher, stronger." *Chemical Engineering News* 77 (1999): 42–52.

38. Bauer, L., Kohlich, A., Hirschwehr, R., et al. "Food allergy: pollen or bee products?" *Journal of Allergy and Clinical Immunology* 97 (1996): 65–73.

39. Remick, D., Chancellor, K., Pederson, J., et al. "Hyperthermia and dehydration-related deaths associated with intentional rapid weight loss in three collegiate wrestlers— North Carolina, Wisconsin, and Michigan, November–December, 1997." *Morbidity and Mortality Weekly Report* 47 (06) (1998): 105–108. Available online at *http://www.cdc.gov/mmwr/preview/mmwrhtml/00051388.htm.*

40. American College of Sports Medicine. "Position stand: Weight loss in wrestlers." *Medicine and Science in Sports and Exercise* 28 (1996): ix–xii.

41. Bennell, K.L., Malcolm, S.A., Wark, J.D., and Brukner, P.D. "Skeletal effects of menstrual disturbances in athletes." *Scandinavian Journal of Medicine and Science in Sports* 7 (1997): 261–273.

42. Beard, J., and Tobin, B. "Iron status and exercise." *American Journal of Clinical Nutrition* 72 (supplement) (2000): 594S–597S.

43. Food and Nutrition Board, Institute of Medicine. *Dietary Reference Intakes: Vitamin A, Vitamin K, Arsenic, Boron, Chromium, Copper, Iodine, Iron, Manganese, Molybdenum, Nickel, Silicon, Vanadium, and Zinc.* Washington, D.C.: National Academy Press, 2001.

44. American College of Sports Medicine. "American College of Sports Medicine position stand: exercise and physical activity for older adults." *Medicine and Science in Sports and Exercise* 30 (1998): 992–1008.

45. U.S. Department of Health and Human Services. "Physical Activity and Health: A Report of the Surgeon General." Centers for Disease Control and Prevention, 1996.

46. U.S. Department of Agriculture, U.S. Department of Health and Human Services. *Nutrition and Your Health: Dietary Guidelines for Americans,* 5th ed. Home and Garden Bulletin, No. 232. Hyattsville, MD: U.S. Government Printing Office, 2000.

47. Andersen, R.E., Crespo, C.J., Bartlett, S.J., et al. "Relationship of physical activity and television watching with body weight and level of fatness among children: Results from the Third National Health and Nutrition Examination Survey." *Journal of the American Medical Association* 279 (1998): 938–942.

Bibliography

American College of Sports Medicine. "American College of Sports Medicine position stand: Exercise and physical activity for older adults." *Medicine and Science in Sports and Exercise* 30 (1998): 992–1008.

———. "Position stand: Weight loss in wrestlers." *Medicine and Science in Sports and Exercise* 28 (1996): ix–xii.

Andersen, R.E., Crespo, C.J., Bartlett, S.J., et al. "Relationship of physical activity and television watching with body weight and level of fatness among children: Results from the Third National Health and Nutrition Examination Survey." *Journal of the American Medical Association* 279 (1998): 938–942.

Armstrong, L.E., and Epstein, Y. "Fluid-electrolyte balance during labor and exercise: concepts and misconceptions." *International Journal of Sport Nutrition* 9 (1999):1–12.

Askew, E.W. "Nutrition and performance in hot, cold, and high-altitude environments," *Nutrition in Exercise and Sport*, 3rd ed., ed. I. Wolinsky. Boca Raton: CRC Press, 1998, pp. 597–619.

Bauer, L., Kohlich, A., Hirschwehr, R., et al. "Food allergy: pollen or bee products?" *Journal of Allergy and Clinical Immunology* 97 (1996): 65–73.

Beard, J., and Tobin, B. "Iron status and exercise." *American Journal of Clinical Nutrition* 72 (supplement) (2000): 594S–597S.

Bennell, K.L., Malcolm, S.A., Wark, J.D., and Brukner, P.D. "Skeletal effects of menstrual disturbances in athletes." *Scandinavian Journal of Medicine and Science in Sports* 7 (1997): 261–273.

Bent, S., Tiedt, T.N., Odden, M.C., and Shlipak, M.G. "The relative safety of ephedra compared with other herbal products." *Annals of Internal Medicine* 138 (2003): 468–471.

Brass, E.P. "Supplemental carnitine and exercise." *American Journal of Clinical Nutrition* 72 (supplement) (2000): 618S–623S.

Bucci, L.R. "Selected herbals and human exercise performance." *American Journal of Clinical Nutrition* 72 (2000): 624S–636S.

Davis, J.M., Welsh, R.S., De Volve, K.L., and Alderson, N.A. "Effects of branched-chain amino acids and carbohydrate on fatigue during intermittent, high-intensity running." *International Journal of Sports Medicine* 20 (1999): 309–314.

Dekkers, J.C., van Doornen, L.J.P., and Kemper, H.C.G. "The role of antioxidant vitamins and enzymes in the prevention of exercise-induced muscle damage." *Sports Medicine* 21 (1996): 213–238.

Dempsey, R.L., Mazzone, M.F., and Meurer, L.N. "Does oral creatine supplementation improve strength? A meta-analysis." *Journal of Family Practice* 1(11) (2001): 945–951.

Feldman, E.B. "Creatine: a dietary supplement and ergogenic aid." *Nutrition Reviews* 57 (1999): 45–50.

Food and Nutrition Board, Institute of Medicine. *Dietary Reference Intakes: Energy, Carbohydrates, Fiber, Fat, Protein, and Amino Acids.* Washington, D.C.: National Academy Press, 2002.

———. *Dietary Reference Intakes: Vitamin A, Vitamin K, Arsenic, Boron, Chromium, Copper, Iodine, Iron, Manganese, Molybdenum, Nickel, Silicon, Vanadium, and Zinc.* Washington, D.C.: National Academy Press, 2001.

Freudenrich, Craig C. "How Exercise Works: Getting the Most from Muscles." Available online at *http://entertainment.howstuffworks.com/sports-physiology6.htm.*

Horowitz, J.F., Mora-Rodriguez, R., Byerley, L.O., and Coyle, E.F. "Pre-exercise medium-chain triglyceride ingestion does not alter muscle glycogen use during exercise." *Journal of Applied Physiology* 88 (1) (2000): 219–225.

JADA. "Nutrition and Athletic Performance—Position of the American Dietetic Association, Dietitians of Canada, and American College of Sports Medicine." *Journal of the American Dietetic Association* 100 (2000): 1543–1556.

Kato, I., Vogelman, J.H., Dilman, V., et al. "Effect of supplementation with chromium picolinate on antibody titers to 5-hydroxymethyl uracil." *European Journal of Epidemiology* 14 (1998): 621–626.

Kreider, R.B., Melton, C., Greenwood, M., et al. "Effects of oral d-ribose supplementation on anaerobic capacity and selected metabolic markers in healthy males." *International Journal of Sport Nutrition and Exercise Metabolism* 13 (1) (2003): 87–96.

Lukaski, H.C. "Chromium as a supplement." *Annual Review of Nutrition* 19 (1999): 279–301.

Manore, M., and Thompson, J. *Sport Nutrition for Health and Performance.* Champaign, IL: Human Kinetics, 2000.

McArdle, W.D., Katch, F.I., and Katch, V.L. *Exercise Physiology: Energy, Nutrition, and Human Performance,* 5th ed. Baltimore: Lippincott Williams & Wilkens, 2001.

Bibliography

Misell, L.M., Lagomarcino, N.D., Schuster, V., and Kern, M. "Chronic medium-chain triacylglycerol consumption and endurance performance in trained runners." *Journal of Sports Medicine and Physical Fitness* 41(2) (2001): 210–215.

Op't Eijnde, B., Van Leemputte, M,. Brouns, F., et al. "No effects of oral ribose supplementation on repeated maximal exercise and de novo ATP resynthesis." *Journal of Applied Physiology* 91(5) (2002): 2275–2281.

Poortmans, J.R., and Francaux, M. "Adverse effects of creatine supplementation: Fact or fiction?" *Sports Medicine* 30 (2000): 155–170.

Quinn, Elizabeth. "Fast and Slow Twitch Muscle Fibers: How They Affect Your Performance." Available online at *http://sportsmedicine.about.com/library/weekly/aa080901a.htm.*

Remick, D., Chancellor, K., Pederson, J., et al. "Hyperthermia and dehydration-related deaths associated with intentional rapid weight loss in three collegiate wrestlers—North Carolina, Wisconsin, and Michigan, November–December, 1997." *Morbidity and Mortality Weekly Report* 47(06) (1998): 105–108. Available online at *http://www.cdc.gov.*

Rhoades, R., and Pflanzer, R. *Human Physiology*, 3rd ed. Philadelphia: Saunders College Publishing, 1996.

Ritter, S.K. "Faster, higher, stronger." *Chemical Engineering News* 77 (1999): 42–52.

"Salt and the Ultraendurance Athlete." Available online at *http://www.rice.edu/~jenky/sports/salt.html.*

Senay, L.C. "Water and electrolytes during physical activity." *Nutrition in Exercise and Sport*, 3rd ed., ed. I. Wolinski. Boca Raton: CRC Press, 1998, pp. 257–276.

Shen, H-P. "Body fluids and water balance." *Biochemical and Physiological Aspects of Human Nutrition*, ed. M. Stipanuk. Philadelphia: W.B. Saunders, 2000, pp. 843–865.

Spriet, L.L. "Caffeine and performance." *International Journal of Sport Nutrition* 5 (supplement) (1995): 84S–99S.

Stearns, D.M., Wise, J.P., Patierno, S.R., and Wetterhahn, K.E. "Chromium (III) picolinate produces damage in Chinese hamster ovary cells." *Federation of American Societies for Experimental Biology Journal* 9 (1995): 1643–1648.

Terjung, R.L., Clarkson, P., Eichner, E.R., et al. "American College of Sports Medicine roundtable: The physiological and health effects of oral creatine supplementation." *Medicine and Science in Sports and Exercise* 32 (2000): 706–717.

U.S. Department of Agriculture, U.S. Department of Health and Human Services. *Nutrition and Your Health: Dietary Guidelines for Americans,* 5th ed. Home and Garden Bulletin, No. 232. Hyattsville, MD: U.S. Government Printing Office, 2000.

U.S. Department of Health and Human Services. "Physical Activity and Health: A Report of the Surgeon General." Centers for Disease Control and Prevention, 1996.

U.S. Food and Drug Administration. Evidence Report/Technology Assessment Number 76. "Ephedra and Ephedrine for Weight Loss and Athletic Performance Enhancement: Clinical Efficacy and Side Effects." Available online at *http://www.fda.gov.*

Van Hall, G., Saris, W.H., van de Schoor, P.A., and Wagenmakers, A.J. "The effect of free glutamine and peptide ingestion on the rate of muscle glycogen resynthesis in man." *International Journal of Sports Medicine* 21 (2000): 25–30.

Williams, M.H. "Facts and fallacies of purported ergogenic amino acid supplements." *Clinical Sports Medicine* 18 (1999): 633–649.

Ziegenfuss, T.N., Berardi, J.M., and Lowery, L.M. "Effects of prohormone supplementation in humans: A review." *Canadian Journal of Applied Physiology* 27(6) (2002): 628–646.

Index

Index

Index

Picture Credits